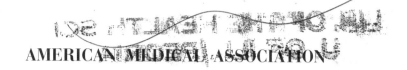

PROFILES OF ADOLESCENT HEALTH SERIES

Volume I # America's Adolescents: How Healthy Are They?

By Janet E. Gans, Ph.D.
in collaboration with

Dale A. Blyth, Ph.D.
Arthur B. Elster, M.D.
Lena Lundgren Gaveras

THE AMA PROFILES OF ADOLESCENT HEALTH SERIES

This is the first volume in a new series that focuses on major issues in adolescent health. The purpose of the AMA Profiles of Adolescent Health is to provide a useful set of references for planning, advocacy, teaching, and community education. The series is intended for people who work with or on behalf of adolescents and who want to know more about the state of their health. Although it provides important information on various topics in adolescent health, the series is not a guide to working with individual adolescents. Each volume in the series is arranged in a question and answer format to enable the reader easily to identify information of greatest interest.

TABLE OF CONTENTS

Chapter 1

How Severe and Widespread Are Adolescent Health Problems?

Chapter 2

What Are Adolescents Doing and Experiencing That Threatens Their Health?

LIST OF FIGURES

LIST OF BOXED INSERTS

EDITORIAL BOARD OF THE AMA PROFILES OF ADOLESCENT HEALTH SERIES

ACKNOWLEDGMENTS

There are many individuals both inside and outside of the American Medical Association who contributed to the success of this volume and the AMA Profiles of Adolescent Health Series more generally. We would first like to thank individuals from government, academic, and social service agencies who offered valuable suggestions about the scope of the series. They include Barbara J. Albertson, M.D., pediatric consultant at the Children's Home and Aid Society of Illinois; Lawrence D'Angelo, M.D., M.P.H., Chairman of the Department of Adolescent and Young Adult Medicine at the Children's National Medical Center; Anthony Dekker, D.O., Director of Adolescent and Young Adult Medicine at Chicago Osteopathic Hospital; Don Dion, M.D., a private practitioner in Indiana; Amy Dinesch, M.A., Executive Director of Planned Parenthood in Chicago; Lonnie Edwards, M.D., former Commissioner of Health in Chicago; Linda Freeman, M.D., a Chicago-based psychiatrist in private practice; Bonnie Jellan, M.H.A., Senior Staff Specialist at the American Hospital Association; Michael Kane, M.S.W., Director of the Response Center; Kathleen Miner, M.A., Executive Director of Southwest YMCA in Alsip, Illinois; Kristin Moore, Ph.D., Senior Research Associate at Child Trends, Inc.; Naomi Morris, M.D., M.P.H., Professor and Director of Community Health Sciences in the School of Public Health at the University of Illinois; Jon Shaw, M.D., formerly of the National Institute of Mental Health; and Gary Strokosch, M.D., Director of the Section of Adolescent Medicine at Rush-Presbyterian-St. Luke's Hospital.

Several individuals provided statistics or other material used in the volume. The authors would like especially to thank Linda Bearinger, R.N., M.S., Instructor of Nursing and Clinic Coordinator at the Adolescent Health Clinic of the University of Minnesota; Richard C. Birkel, Ph.D., formerly Director of the Office of Prevention at the National Mental Health Association; Michael Cohen, M.D., Chairman of the Department of Pediatrics at Montefiore Medical Center; Gayle Geber, M.P.H., Program Director at the National Center for Youth With Disabilities; Kay Johnson, M.P.H., M.Ed., Director, Health Division at the Children's Defense Fund; Elizabeth R. McAnarney, M.D., Director of the Division of General Pediatrics at the University of Rochester; Margaret A. McManus, M.H.S., President of McManus Health Policy, Inc.; Paul W. Newacheck, Dr.P.H., Associate Professor at the Institute for Health Policy Studies at the University of California-San Francisco; John E. Schowalter, M.D., Albert J. Solnit Professor of

Child Psychiatry and Pediatrics at the Yale Child Study Center at Yale University and President of the American Academy of Child and Adolescent Psychiatry; Sheri Scott, M.P.H., Project Coordinator for the Promoting Healthy Traditions program at the American Indian Health Care Association; and the Alan Guttmacher Institute, which allowed us to use copyrighted material. Robert W. Blum, M.D., M.P.H., Ph.D., Director of the Adolescent Health Program and Associate Professor of Pediatrics and Maternal and Child Health at the University of Minnesota; Joy Dryfoos, a private consultant; Alex Gralnick, M.D., Medical Director of High Point Hospital; and Michael D. Resnick, Ph.D., Associate Professor and Director of Research and Demonstration Programs Adolescent Health Program, School of Public Health at the University of Minnesota, also provided useful suggestions during the development of the volume.

This volume would not have been possible without the continued support and encouragement of William R. Hendee, Ph.D., Vice President for Science and Technology, and Robert C. Rinaldi, Director of the Division of Health Sciences, both of the American Medical Association. Other colleagues at the American Medical Association helped make this volume useful to physicians and other health professionals working with or on behalf of adolescents. The authors appreciate the careful reviews provided by Roger L. Brown, Ph.D., Missy Fleming, Ph.D., John J. Henning, Ph.D., Randall L. Morrison, Ph.D., Marshall D. Rosman, Ph.D., Katherine H. Voetgle, Ph.D., and Bonnie B. Wilford, M.A.

Kelly Carafotas and Yolanda Davis deserve special thanks for their tireless and far-flung search for statistics. Many thanks to Kelly Koski for her thorough and creative work on the index. Nicole Netter did a terrific editorial job and the volume has benefited greatly from her red pen. Mary F. Kizer and Linda Blyth also played an invaluable role in helping to prepare the manuscript for final publication. Finally, our special thanks to Donna McGrath, Sharna Fetman, Michaelene Brown, Rhonda Taira, and David Doty, who were particularly helpful in turning the manuscript into an attractive and visually appealing book.

EXECUTIVE SUMMARY

America's Adolescents: How Healthy Are They?
Volume One in the *AMA Profiles of Adolescent Health Series*

As the year 2000 approaches, many adolescents in the United States will experience problems that threaten not only their current health but also their ability to become healthy adults capable of leading full, productive lives. The American Medical Association has long been concerned about adolescent health and how it can be improved. The task is complex because many adolescent health problems are intimately linked with educational performance, family relationships, poverty, and the general lifestyles that adolescents experience in their communities.

Although serious, chronic medical and psychiatric disorders affect approximately 2 million adolescents (6% of the adolescent population), many more adolescents today are at risk for death and other poor health outcomes that are not primarily biomedical in origin. Contemporary threats to adolescent health, the so-called "social morbidities," are primarily the result of social environment and/or behavior. Social morbidities include suicide, homicide, substance abuse, sexually transmitted diseases (STDs), unintended pregnancy, and the human immunodeficiency virus (HIV) infection that can lead to acquired immunodeficiency syndrome (AIDS).

Medical and social science research on adolescents has revealed two disturbing trends. First, many health problems are affecting adolescents at younger ages. For example, the decline in age at first intercourse (and delay in contraceptive use by young sexually active adolescents) has produced increased rates of sexually transmitted disease among adolescents. Gonorrhea rates are actually higher among sexually active 15- to 19-year-olds than among 20- to 24-year-olds. More adolescents are also experimenting with harmful substances at younger ages. For example, between the 1950s and the 1980s the percentage of students who had ever tried an illicit substance prior to the 10th grade rose from less than 5% to 30%. A second disturbing trend is the simultaneous involvement of youth in several health-threatening behaviors, such as drug use, delinquency, unprotected sex, and sex with many partners. Approximately 25% of adolescents lead "high-risk" lifestyles that result in injury, hospitalization, or other unhealthy consequences.

Of course, most adolescents do not lead dangerous lives but neither do they take precautions to ensure good health, such as getting adequate nutrition and exercise. More than half of adolescents do not use seat belts, and 44% report riding in an automobile with a driver who has been drinking or using drugs.

The AMA recognizes that in order to plan effective prevention and intervention strategies that will ensure a healthy transition to adulthood, it is important to understand the prevalence and severity of adolescent health problems, the groups of adolescents who are most affected by particular health threats, and the areas in which adolescent health has improved or deteriorated. The following facts highlight the health status of adolescents in terms of violence, injury, and abuse; substance use; sexuality; HIV/AIDS; mental health and disorders; and general physical health.

Violence, Injury, and Abuse

- Violence and injury account for three of four adolescent deaths. More than 3 of 10 adolescents who die are killed in a motor vehicle accident, and half of these accidents involve alcohol.

- The homicide rate has doubled among 10- to 14-year-olds during the past 20 years. Homicide is the leading cause of death among black 15- to 19-year-olds.

- Over the past 20 years the suicide rate tripled among 10- to 14-year-olds and doubled among 15- to 19-year-olds. Whites are 3 times more likely than blacks to die of suicide.

- Abuse and neglect increased 74% during the past decade, and adolescents experience more abuse and neglect than younger children do. Consequences of abuse include depression, insomnia, and other psychological difficulties during adolescence and adulthood.

Substance Use

- Ninety-two percent of high school seniors have consumed alcohol at least once, 50% have tried marijuana, and 15% have tried cocaine. Although drug use is often considered an adolescent problem, experimentation frequently begins before adolescence, and use of some substances is more prevalent among young adults 18 to 25 years of age.

- White adolescents are more likely than black or Hispanic adolescents to experiment with alcohol, tobacco, and most other drugs. They are also more likely to become heavy users of all harmful substances except alcohol.

- Substance use proceeds in stages. Tobacco, alcohol, or marijuana can be "gateway drugs," substances that may lead to the use of other drugs. Adolescents who currently drink alcohol are 10 times more likely than nondrinkers to use marijuana and 11 times more likely to use cocaine.

- Since the late 1970s there has been a decline among adolescents in cigarette smoking and in the use of most illicit drugs. During this time there was a dramatic increase in the perceived harmfulness of illicit drugs reported by adolescents.

Sexuality

- By the time they are 18 years old, 65% of boys and 51% of girls are sexually active. Approximately 50% of American adolescents do not use contraceptives the first time they have intercourse. Half of premarital pregnancies occur within the first 6 months after sexual initiation. Eleven percent of adolescent women become pregnant each year, and 4% have an abortion.

- Adolescents who get pregnant while in high school are more likely to drop out of school, become dependent on welfare, and become single parents.

- Between 1950 and 1985 the nonmarital birth rate among adolescents younger than 20 years of age increased 300% for whites and 16% for blacks. Approximately 2.5 million adolescents have had a sexually transmitted disease, and one in four sexually active adolescents will contract an STD before graduating from high school. Sexually transmitted disease rates are substantially higher among black than white adolescents.

HIV/AIDS

- More than two of three adolescents with AIDS were infected through sexual contact with adults. Although only 440 people with AIDS (fewer than 1%) are between 13 and 19 years of age, the prevalence of HIV infection among adolescents is a source of concern. Because it takes an estimated 5 to 10 years for the HIV infection to result in AIDS, many young adults who have AIDS contracted the virus as adolescents. Approximately 20% of people identified as having AIDS are between 20 and 29 years of age.

Mental Health and Disorders

- Alcohol and drug abuse, suicide, homicide, and other health problems that occur among adolescents are frequently considered symptoms of psychological distress.

- Mental disorders affect 634,000 adolescents and account for 32% of disabilities among 10- to 18-year-olds.

- It is estimated that 5 million children and adolescents need mental health services but do not receive them.

- The 10% increase in the psychiatric hospitalization of adolescents during the past decade has generated controversy over the appropriate array of psychological treatments available to adolescents.

General Physical Health

- Children in poverty are in poorer health and are significantly less likely to have health insurance than are children in families with annual incomes over $35,000.

- Approximately 5% of adolescents are obese, and as many as 25% are overweight. Between 1% and 2% of adolescents have persistent hypertension, a condition linked to heart disease and stroke in adults.

These health problems offer ample cause for concern, but they are not insurmountable. Through appropriate prevention and intervention efforts, improvements in adolescent health can occur. Improvements in access to and use of health services are part of the answer. Today there are several noteworthy programs and initiatives taking place in communities and in organized medicine.

It is imperative that such efforts are responsive to demographic changes in the adolescent population. Over the next 10 years, increasing numbers of adolescents will come from economically disadvantaged and minority backgrounds. As the year 2000 approaches it is critical that government, business, foundations, community groups, schools, organized medicine, and other interested groups cooperate and coordinate activities to promote adolescent health and well-being, thereby ensuring that each young person has an opportunity to contribute to and share in the nation's prosperity and reach his or her potential.

INTRODUCTION

The second decade of life has always been a time of rapid physical growth and development. It is often a challenging and confusing time for adolescents, their families, teachers, health providers, and others in the community who live and work with them. Today's adolescents experience health problems that threaten not only their current health but also their ability to become healthy adults capable of leading full, productive lives. Business leaders and educators agree that the labor force of the future will need educated, healthy adults if the United States is to remain competitive in the global economy. The widespread availability of illicit drugs, increased pressures for sexual intimacy, decreased levels of social support, and increased ambiguity over their roles in society have made the transition from childhood to adulthood more difficult for adolescents than ever before.

Society has a moral obligation to ensure the health and well-being of all children and adolescents. Adolescents' families are different than they were in the past. Since 1950 the number of children each year involved in divorces has quadrupled. In 1985, 21% of children lived in single-parent families (113). Today, one of every five American children younger than 18 lives in poverty, and children from racial and ethnic minorities are overrepresented among the poor. These youth are more likely to experience violence, abuse and neglect, and injury. These realities are cause for concern because in the future an increasing proportion of adolescents will come from minority families or live in poverty.

The adolescent population in the United States is changing in size and composition. In 1985 there were more than 35 million 10- to 19-year-olds in the United States (78). By 1990 the adolescent population will decline to 33.8 million and then increase to 38.5 million by the year 2000. In 2000, the adolescent population will be younger than it is today (disproportionately comprised of 10- to 14-year-olds) and include a greater proportion of racial and ethnic minorities. In 1985 close to 27% of adolescents belonged to racial and ethnic minority groups; by 2000, black, Asian, Hispanic, and Native American adolescents will constitute 31% of adolescents, with the greatest increase among Hispanics and Asians. In many cities and a few states, minority groups will be the emergent majority. These changes underscore the need for society to ensure that the transition into adolescence is healthy and responsive to the needs of diverse racial and ethnic groups.

The American Medical Association has long been concerned about adolescent health. In hospitals, emergency rooms, physicians' offices, health maintenance organizations (HMOs), community health clinics, and school-based health centers, physicians treat adolescents who are pregnant, who have sexually transmitted diseases, who are injured in car accidents, who are suicidal or failing in school, and who shoot drugs and are shot with guns. They see adolescents who eat too many of the wrong foods, who starve themselves, or who are obese or get insufficient exercise. These unhealthy behaviors can result in reduced life expectancy, cancer, heart disease, stroke, developmental delays, or psychological problems. Many of these problems can be prevented, and the human and financial toll on society can be reduced. The AMA believes strongly that providing information about the nature and scope of health problems among adolescents is an essential part of developing effective strategies for solving them. AMA policy recommendations on various issues affecting adolescent health are included in this volume.

The purpose of this volume is to provide an overview of major issues in adolescent health. Chapter 1 examines the prevalence and severity of adolescent health problems and whether adolescents receive the health services they need. In some respects adolescents are a very healthy population, but for all too many, their environment and behavior often pose serious health risks. Chapter 2 describes how violence, physical and sexual abuse, drug use (including use of tobacco and alcohol), and sexual activity threaten the well-being of adolescents. Chapter 3 reviews trends in adolescent health: how it has improved and how it has gotten worse. Chapter 4 identifies the degree to which adolescents are at risk for various health threats depending on their age, race, sex, and family income. Chapter 5 describes efforts by public and private groups and suggests items for organized medicine's agenda to improve adolescent health.

Terminology Used in This Volume

Adolescence can be divided into different age groups, each of which reflects a different biopsychosocial stage of development. In general, throughout this volume, "early" or "young adolescents" refers to people between the ages of 10 and 14 years of age. "Older adolescents" refers to 15- to 19-year-olds, and "young adults" refers to those who are approximately 18 to 24 years of age. The terms "girls" and "boys" are used to refer to adolescents who are younger than 15, while "men" and "women" refer to adolescents who are 15 years of age or older.

Some Limitations of Data on Adolescent Health

Research on adolescents is growing but remains incomplete and somewhat problematic. For example, age categories differ from one study to the next, and adolescents are often combined into an age category with either children or adults. Whenever possible, data presented in this volume refer to the 10- to 19-year-old age range or specific subgroups of that age range. Sometimes inconsistencies between surveys have resulted in age groupings that include children or young adults. At times this complicates getting a clear picture of the health problems and needs of adolescents as a distinct age group. These problems can be minimized as researchers reach greater consensus about appropriate and relevant age groupings for adolescents.

There are also other limitations in available data on adolescents. In many instances, data are unavailable for Hispanics, various groups of Asian Americans, or Native Americans. Frequently, too, data on family income are not available, making it difficult to determine whether health problems are primarily due to socioeconomic or racial or ethnic differences. Data on mental health and disorders are sketchy, and trend data are not available on many adolescent mental health issues, limiting the depth of discussion possible on this topic. The data in this volume are drawn primarily from reliable national surveys, though in rare instances data from regional, state, or local samples have been cited. The most current data available at the time of publication have been incorporated wherever possible.

1.

How severe and widespread are adolescent health problems?

Overall, the majority of adolescents appear to be relatively healthy in traditional medical terms, with low rates of cancer, hypertension, heart disease, and other physical disorders. When viewed more broadly in terms of risk-taking behavior and emotional health, however, adolescents experience a number of problems that threaten their overall health and well-being. Some of these health problems are more serious than others. This chapter examines the prevalence and severity of medical conditions affecting adolescents, beginning with the most disabling conditions. Important but less debilitating conditions that can disrupt adolescents' lives on either a short-term or a long-term basis are also noted. The chapter then reviews access to and use of health services by adolescents, which are key to detecting physical or emotional complications of rapid growth and development. The prevalence and severity of adolescents' mental health problems are also addressed, and limitations of data on this topic are noted. A review of the leading causes of death illustrates the strong and most obvious links between adolescent mental health and physical well-being.

The questions addressed in this chapter are:

1. What are the more important physiological health problems of adolescents?

2. Are adolescents getting the health care they need?

3. How psychologically and emotionally healthy are today's adolescents?

4. What are the leading causes of death among today's adolescents?

1. What are the more important physiological health problems of adolescents?

Like all age groups, adolescents experience a variety of chronic and acute health problems, some more serious than others. A chronic condition lasts for a prolonged time (at least 3 months) or recurs from time to time. Asthma, diabetes, allergies, and cancer are examples of chronic conditions. An acute condition is one that appears suddenly and is of short duration but severe enough to involve contact with a physician. Strep throat, influenza, and urinary tract infections are examples of acute conditions.

What is it like for families with disabled adolescents?

Adolescents with disabilities face special challenges, as do their families. A survey of 25 learning-disabled young adults reported that 85% were teased by their peers when they were adolescents, 68% felt rejected by peers or family members, and 23% reported that they did not have friends (125). A national survey reported that 10% of families with a disabled child have severe problems making ends meet financially, 5% of parents quit or changed jobs, and 2% of couples divorced because of their child's condition (62). A survey of families with disabled children reported that the average annual expenditures for hospital and physician expenses ranged from $870 to $10,299 for a disabled child, compared with $270 for a nondisabled child (83).

Many adolescents have chronic, disabling medical conditions serious enough to prevent or disrupt normal daily activities, such as going to school or participating in sports or other recreational pursuits. Other adolescents have more common and generally less disabling medical conditions, some of which are related to rapid physical growth during adolescence. The severity and prevalence of disabling conditions and illness among adolescents are reviewed here.

About 2 million adolescents aged 10 to 18 (6%) have a serious chronic condition that limits their activity (93).

About 4% of these noninstitutionalized adolescents were limited in the kind or amount of major activity, and 0.5% (165,000 adolescents) were unable to conduct a major activity such as going to school (93).

Adolescents with disabilities spend over 3 times more days in bed than adolescents without disabilities (93).

Adolescents with disabilities face major problems with transitions into and out of adolescence. These include transitions into adult sexuality, independent living, employment, and moving into the adult health care system. Although faced by all adolescents, these transitions are especially difficult for disabled youth because of their complex health needs and limitations on the types of employment and level of independence they are able to attain (29).

Causes of Disability Among 10- to 18-Year-Olds

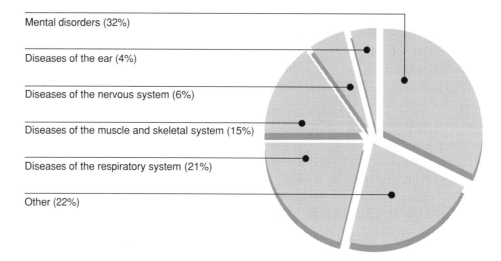

Mental disorders (32%)

Diseases of the ear (4%)

Diseases of the nervous system (6%)

Diseases of the muscle and skeletal system (15%)

Diseases of the respiratory system (21%)

Other (22%)

Source: 1984 Health Interview Survey data, in Newacheck, P. W. (1989). Adolescents with special health needs: Prevalence, severity, and access to health services. *Pediatrics, 84,* 872-881.

AMA Profiles of Adolescent Health

Causes of Disability

■ As noted in the chart, there are five leading causes of disability among 10- to 18-year-olds (93).

• The leading chronic disabilities are mental disorders, including psychoses, anxiety and personality disorders, substance dependence syndromes, and mental retardation. These affect an estimated 634,000 adolescents (93).

• Chronic respiratory conditions affect 406,000 adolescents and include asthma, bronchitis, and various other conditions of the respiratory tract (93).

• Diseases of the muscle and skeletal system and connective tissue, including arthritis, other disorders of the joints and bones, and other deformities, affect 295,000 adolescents (93).

• Diseases of the nervous system, such as multiple sclerosis, cerebral palsy, epilepsy, and other degenerative or hereditary disorders of the central nervous system, affect 115,000 adolescents (93).

• Diseases related to the ear affect an estimated 80,000 adolescents and consist mostly of deafness and other hearing impairments (93).

• The other 22% of leading disabilities includes a variety of disorders, such as diseases of the digestive system, urinary system, blood and blood-forming organs, eye disorders, heart disease, rheumatic fever, tumors, venereal disease, viral diseases, and bacterial diseases (93).

Other Chronic Conditions

Many adolescents have less debilitating but important medical conditions that can interfere with their lives on either a short-term or a long-term basis.

Between 1% and 2% of adolescents have persistent hypertension (high blood pressure), a condition linked to heart disease and stroke in adults (108).

For about 5% of adolescents, rapid and uneven skeletal growth results in scoliosis (curvature of the spine). Although scoliosis is often not severe, one in 1,000 youth requires treatment with a brace or surgery to keep the curvature from getting worse (38).

Dysmenorrhea (pain or discomfort associated with menstruation) affects almost half of all female adolescents and is a leading cause of episodic school absenteeism (70).

Myopia (nearsightedness) usually appears around puberty; the rate increases progressively until the early 20s when it stabilizes. About 25% of 12- to 17-year-olds are nearsighted (75).

About 5% of adolescents in the United States are obese (i.e., more than 20% over the maximum recommended weight for their height) (75), and between 5% and 25% are overweight (38).

- Almost 80% of obese adolescents will be obese adults and suffer physical, psychological, and social disadvantages associated with obesity (38).

- Obesity and being overweight can lead to hypertension, increased cholesterol levels, diabetes, and reduced life expectancy (75).

Only 4% of high school students are free of any dental decay (75), and 23% of adolescents age 15 have untreated decay on at least one tooth surface (118).

Serious malocclusion, the lack of good contact between the upper and lower jaw when closed, affects 50% of adolescents and often requires braces (75).

Gum disease increases dramatically between the ages of 12 and 17 and may be due to hormonal changes during puberty (75).

Reasons Adolescents Seek Care

Another way to gauge the nature of adolescent health problems is to examine the reasons adolescents seek care. Almost half of all office visits with physicians cannot easily be classified because they reflect a wide array of specific problems, each of which accounts for fewer than 2% of visits (46).

- Among 11- to 14-year-old boys, general medical examinations and preparticipation athletic exams account for 12% of physician visits, coughs and other throat problems account for 9% of visits, and skin and cosmetic problems, such as rashes, acne, and warts, prompt 6% of visits to physicians (46).

- Similar proportions of 11- to 14-year-old boys and girls visit physicians for preventive health examinations (11%) or skin and cosmetic problems (6%), but girls have a higher percentage of visits for coughs and throat problems (15%) than boys do (9%) (46).

- Regardless of sex, 15- to 20-year-olds have half as many preventive health care visits to private physicians than their younger counterparts (46).

- For 15- to 20-year-old men, skin and cosmetic problems account for the largest proportion (12%) of physician visits. Other reasons for visits are similar to those of younger adolescent boys (46).

- For 15- to 20-year-old women, prenatal care accounts for 14% of physician visits. Other reasons for visits are similar to those of younger adolescent girls (46).

Good health is necessary for adolescents to learn in school. Poor vision, discomfort, weakness, or fatigue from undiagnosed or untreated medical conditions can interfere with the ability to concentrate and process educational material.

2. Are adolescents getting the health care they need?

Compared to adults, adolescents have fewer chronic conditions, fewer short-term hospital stays, and fewer days when they stay home sick in bed. They are also more likely to be assessed in excellent or very good health (1). It is important, however, that adolescents receive proper screening during puberty in order to detect physical and emotional disorders related to rapid physical and hormonal changes and to manage chronic disorders properly. Despite these facts, there is evidence that many adolescents may not get the health care they need. The availability of health services and whether adolescents seek the services they need are complicated by many factors. Because many adolescents do not receive needed health services, alternative service delivery models have been developed in schools, correctional institutions, and freestanding comprehensive health clinics.

In 1981 the Select Panel for the Promotion of Child Health reported that 14% of children and adolescents under the age of 18 do not receive the medical care they need (105).

In 1980-1981, adolescents 11 to 20 years of age comprised 17% of the population but only 11% of visits to physicians' offices (64).

Over 70% of visits for health care by adolescents are to private physicians. Twelve percent of adolescents have no regular source of care (105).

In 1988 about 30% of adolescents between the ages of 12 and 17 had not seen a physician during the past year, compared to 10% of children under the age of 4 and 16% of children 5 to 7 years of age (1).

On the average, adolescents between the ages of 12 and 17 have fewer physician contacts per year than younger children (3.2 visits compared to 6.1 visits) (1).

At least 7.5 million children under the age of 18 (12%) are in need of some type of mental health services, but fewer than one third of those youth actually receive treatment (103).

Pregnant adolescents are less likely than women in other age groups to obtain early prenatal care, and they are most likely to receive late or no prenatal care (61).

- Of babies born to adolescents in 1985, 53% had mothers who received care in the first 3 months of pregnancy, compared to 76% of babies born to women of all ages (61).

- In 1985, 6% of babies were born to women who received late or no care, compared to 12% of babies born to adolescent women (61).

Public attitudes favor health services for adolescents

The majority of Americans support the availability of health services for adolescents and believe that they should be funded by the government. A 1987 AMA survey found that 69% of the public agreed that there was a need for a clinic in their community that provides health services to adolescents for problems, such as alcohol, drug abuse, mental health, sexual problems, and birth control. Sixty-five percent thought that such clinics should be funded by federal, state, or local government. Nineteen percent thought that funding should come from private sources (56).

Barriers to Health Services

Barriers to health services for adolescents include:

- lack of insurance coverage or money to cover charges independent of parents;

- office hours that conflict with school schedules;

- discomfort with various health care settings;

- requirements for parental consent;

- perceived or actual lack of confidentiality between adolescents and their health providers;

- inability or failure to comply with a provider's instructions or follow up on referral recommendations (7).

The lack of insurance has a major effect on whether or not adolescents receive health services and the frequency of services received (94).

- Adolescents without health insurance wait longer periods of time between physician visits. Adolescents who last saw a physician 2 years ago are more than twice as likely to be uninsured than adolescents who saw a physician during the past year (94).

- A total of 4.5 million adolescents in the United States (14%) are without any form of private or public (i.e., Medicaid) health insurance coverage (94).

- Uninsured adolescents are concentrated in families that are poor or near poor, have little formal education, and are minorities, particularly Hispanics (94).

- Among uninsured adolescents who live with a parent, approximately half live with a full-year, full-time worker (71).

School-Based Health Centers

In order to increase access to care, attention has focused on using the school setting for health centers. There are currently more than 120 school-based health centers that provide services to adolescents who might not otherwise receive such care (7).

- The success of school-based health centers reflects in part their flexibility, parent support, easy access, no cost or low cost to students, partnership with school staff and community services, and student involvement (72).

- Controversy surrounding school-based health centers revolves around issues of reproduction, including counseling and the distribution of contraceptive devices or prescriptions. However, only 20% of total visits to school-based health programs are for family planning services (7).

Almost 9 of 10 (87%) physicians report that they would refer adolescents to a clinic devoted strictly to adolescent health services (56).

A majority of physicians (63%) believe 15- to 17-year-olds should be able to consult a physician privately without parents being informed of the nature or outcome of the visit. Thirty-nine percent approve of 12- to 14-year-olds visiting physicians without parents being informed (56).

Alternative Health Services

In addition to school-based health centers, alternative health service delivery models are needed for hard-to-reach adolescents who are not in school (e.g., homeless, runaway, or incarcerated youth). Special community or institution-based health services are critical.

The 53,500 youth incarcerated in correctional institutions represent a vastly underserved population with greater than average health care needs. Many have underlying, undiagnosed, or untreated physical and emotional disorders, and most

---

Highlights of AMA policy recommendations on school-based health centers

The AMA recognizes the promise of school-based health centers to provide health services to adolescents, particularly in medically underserved areas. Where school-based health services exist, they should meet the following minimum standards: (a) Health services in schools must be supervised by a physician, preferably one who is experienced in the care of children and adolescents. Additionally, a physician should be accessible to administer care on a regular basis. (b) On-site services should be provided by a professionally prepared school nurse or similarly qualified health professional. Expertise in child and adolescent development, psychosocial and behavioral problems, and emergency care is desirable. Responsibilities of this professional would include coordinating the health care of students with the student, the parents, the school, and the student's personal physician, and assisting with the development and presentation of health education programs in the classroom. (c) There should be a written policy to govern provision of health services in the school, developed by a school health council consisting of school and community-based physicians and nurses, school faculty and administrators, parents and (as appropriate) students, community leaders, and others. (d) Before patient services begin, policies on confidentiality should be established with the advice of expert legal advisors and the school health council. (e) Policies for ongoing monitoring, quality assurance, and evaluation should be established and executed. (f) Health care services should be available during school hours. During other hours an appropriate referral system should be instituted. (g) School-based health programs should draw on outside resources for care, such as private practitioners, public health and mental health clinics, and mental health and neighborhood health programs. (h) Services provided should be coordinated to ensure comprehensive care. Parents should be encouraged to be intimately involved in the health supervision and education of their children (7).

lack a coordinated source of regular health care (8).

- Of juveniles in custody, 63% used drugs regularly prior to their incarceration, 32% were under the influence of alcohol when they committed their offense, and 39% were under the influence of another drug (79).

- Past or present symptoms that meet diagnostic criteria for major depression have been found in approximately 20% of juveniles in correctional facilities (51, 74).

While youth are confined in correctional facilities, they should be protected as much as possible from developing physical and emotional problems as a result of incarceration (8).

This group of disenfranchised youth should receive appropriate health care intervention to help them become more productive citizens (8).

3. How psychologically and emotionally healthy are today's adolescents?

Psychological and physical health are closely intertwined. Alcohol and drug abuse, suicide, homicide, and other health problems that occur at alarming rates among adolescents (see chapter 2) are frequently considered symptoms of psychological distress. Unfortunately, uniform and reliable national prevalence estimates of mental distress and disorders among adolescents do not exist. Instead, a variety of evidence must be used to construct a profile of adolescent mental health. Useful indicators in addition to those already mentioned include self-reported depression and coping difficulties, visits for psychological counseling, and psychiatric hospitalization.

Sex differences in suicide and reported depression

There are important sex differences in attempted and completed suicide. Adolescent girls are 4 to 5 times more likely than boys to attempt suicide, but boys are 4 times more likely than girls to die of suicide, mainly because they choose more lethal methods (28). Girls typically use pills when attempting suicide, while boys tend to use firearms or hanging (75).

A recent survey of 8th and 10th graders found that girls are twice as likely as boys to report feeling sad and hopeless and feel they have nothing to look forward to (19). This result is consistent with the clinical literature, which shows that females have higher rates of depression than males during both adolescence and adulthood (102).

Adolescents Reporting Coping Difficulties and Depression

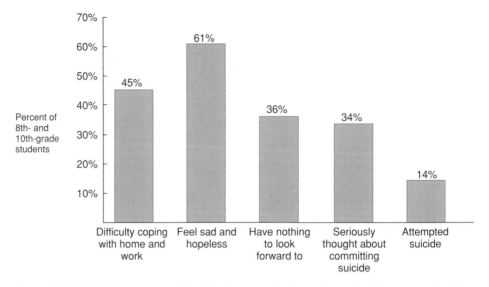

Source: 1987 NASHS data, in American School Health Association, Association for the Advancement of Health Education, & Society for Public Health Education, Inc. (1989). *The National Adolescent Student Health Survey: A report on the health of America's youth.* Oakland, CA: Third Party Publishing.

AMA Profiles of Adolescent Health

In a 1988 Gallup poll, 85% of adolescents said that they were satisfied with their personal lives (26).

However, as noted in the chart above, when 8th- and 10th-grade students were asked specific questions about their feelings, many reported having coping difficulties and suicide attempts (19).

- Sixty-one percent of 8th and 10th graders report feeling depressed and hopeless (19).

- Forty-five percent report having trouble coping with stressful situations at home and school (19).

- Thirty-six percent feel they often or sometimes have nothing to look forward to (19).

- Thirty-four percent have considered committing suicide, and 14% have attempted suicide (19).

It is estimated that for every completed suicide there are between 50 and 200 attempted suicides (75).

One of three homosexual and bisexual boys have attempted suicide. Homosexual youth are 2 to 3 times more likely to attempt suicide than other young people. They comprise approximately 30% of completed youth suicides annually (99).

In 1981, an estimated 1.9 million 12- to 17-year-olds (9%) had received psychological counseling at some point in their lives; 4% had received psychological help within the last year (126).

Divorce and family disruption can create great psychological distress for adolescents. Fourteen percent of adolescents in mother-only families or mother-stepfather families received psychological help at some point in their lives, compared to 5% of adolescents living with both biological parents (126).

Serious psychological problems sometimes go undetected because parents, teachers, and other professionals assume that major mood swings, changes in friendship groups, and wide variation in school grades are normal parts of adolescence, rather than indications of underlying emotional problems.

Psychological disorders that generally have their onset during adolescence include (103):

- anxiety disorders of adolescence (e.g., avoidant disorder);

- schizophrenic disorders of adolescence;

- eating disorders (anorexia nervosa, bulimia);

- substance use disorders (alcohol or drug abuse or multiple drug use).

Social phobias generally have their onset during early adolescence, whereas schizophrenic disorders, panic disorders, and obsessive-compulsive disorders generally have their onset during late adolescence (103).

It is difficult to estimate accurately the number of adolescents with serious eating disorders both because large population-based studies have not been done and because definitions of eating disorders vary considerably among surveys. Estimates suggest that between 5% and 12% of adolescents have an eating disorder. Eating disorders are more common among females than males and occur more frequently among middle- and upper-income than lower-income youth (22, 92).

In 1986 more than 115,000 youth under the age of 18 (less than 1%) were admitted to a psychiatric hospital. Half were admitted to a general hospital psychiatric unit, 36% to a private psychiatric hospital, and 13% to a state hospital (91). Trends and controversies in the psychiatric hospitalization of adolescents are discussed in chapter 3.

4. What are the leading causes of death among today's adolescents?

Some of today's adolescents will not live to adulthood. Most of these deaths will result from violence or injury and could, therefore, be prevented. Death statistics are important indicators of adolescent mental health and risk-taking behavior as well as the nature of the society in which they live.

If 1985 death rates persist, 55 of every 100,000 adolescents will die. This translates into more than 19,800 deaths a year, or 54 deaths each day (49).

◼ As indicated in the pie chart, 10- to 19-year-olds die of several causes (49).

• More than 3 of every 10 adolescents who die are killed in a motor vehicle accident (49), and

half of these accidents involve alcohol (86).

• About 1 in 10 adolescent deaths is due to homicide (49). The homicide rate among black adolescents is especially high. (Details appear in chapter 4.)

• One in 10 deaths among 10- to 19-year-olds is due to suicide (49). Trends showing the dramatic increase in suicide appear in chapter 3, and important age and sex differences in adolescent suicide appear in chapter 4.

• One in 10 adolescent deaths is due to some other violent act or injury (49).

• Violence and injury account for three of every four adolescent deaths (49).

Causes of Death Among 10- to 19-Year-Olds

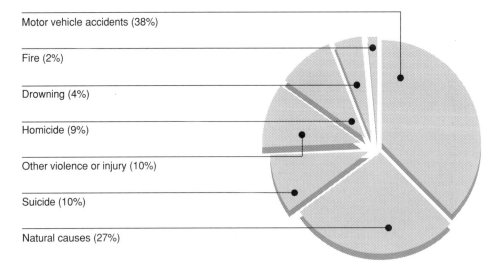

Motor vehicle accidents (38%)

Fire (2%)

Drowning (4%)

Homicide (9%)

Other violence or injury (10%)

Suicide (10%)

Natural causes (27%)

Source: 1983-85, in Fingerhut, L. A., & Kleinman, J. C. (1989). *Trends and current status in childhood mortality, United States, 1900-85*. Vital and Health Statistics, Series 3, No. 26 (DHHS Publication No. PHS 89-1410). Hyattsville, MD: National Center for Health Statistics.

AMA Profiles of Adolescent Health

• Fewer than 3 of 10 adolescent deaths are from natural causes. Malignant tumors and birth defects account for half of these deaths (49).

In 1985, approximately . . .

• 7,503 adolescents 10 to 19 years of age died in motor vehicle accidents;

• 1,850 were victims of homicide;

• 2,130 committed suicide;

• 3,210 died of some other violence or injury;

• 5,377 died of natural causes (49).

Approximately 40 adolescents died each day in 1985 from violence or injury.

Over the past 50 years, the leading causes of death have shifted from natural causes to injury and violence (see chapter 3) (49).

Summary and Implications

Although some adolescents have serious chronic illnesses, modern medical science and public health efforts have reduced the prevalence and fatality of many diseases and illnesses among adolescents. Health threats to today's youth are rooted primarily in psychosocial rather than natural causes. Millions of adolescents do not receive needed physical or mental health services, which places them in short-term and long-term jeopardy. The lack of services places adolescents at risk for a variety of minor and more serious health problems and can disrupt their education, achievement, and productivity as adults. Significant numbers of youth have difficulty coping with stresses in their lives, and thousands die each year of preventable causes. Future improvements in adolescent health are unlikely to come without major health prevention and promotion efforts, along with family and community services that change behavior and experiences.

Chapter

2.

What are adolescents doing and experiencing that threatens their health?

The health of many adolescents is threatened by their environment and lifestyles, though the nature and severity of risk varies among them. Some adolescents live in communities or lead lifestyles characterized by violence, delinquency, substance abuse, and sexual promiscuity. These youth are at high risk for a variety of poor health outcomes, including suicide, drug overdose, hepatitis, accidents and injuries, and sexually transmitted disease. Also at high risk are adolescents who are victimized by adults, through abuse or neglect.

There are other adolescents who lead drug-free and abstinent or sexually responsible lives, who respect authority, and who are surrounded by caring adults. Some of these youth may still be at risk because of poor or inadequate nutritional habits, insufficient exercise, or not engaging in health-promoting activities such as wearing seat belts. For the most part, however, they will not experience the serious health threats described above. Overall, the majority of adolescents engage in some risk-taking behavior but do not experience tragic consequences.

Recent research findings suggest that the age at which adolescents first experiment with sex, tobacco, alcohol, and other drugs is important. Adolescents who begin experimenting with health-compromising behaviors at a young age are more likely to get heavily involved in these activities and experience negative short-term and long-term consequences. For this reason it is important to consider the age at which substance use and sexual activity begins in addition to the prevalence of these activities among adolescents.

This chapter reviews health threats in adolescents' lives, both as victims of others' behavior and as victims of their own behavior.

The questions addressed in this chapter are:

1. **How widespread are violence and abuse in adolescents' lives?**

2. **How prevalent are tobacco, alcohol, and drug use among today's adolescents?**

3. **How many adolescents are sexually active and how does this threaten their health?**

4. **In what other ways do adolescents' lifestyles place them at risk?**

1. How widespread are violence and abuse in adolescents' lives?

The lives of many adolescents are characterized by a high degree of violence, injury, abuse, and neglect. Adolescents confront violence and abuse in many environments traditionally viewed as safe havens—at home, among peers, and in the community. Furthermore, adolescents commit a disproportionate amount of violent crimes and many hold attitudes that encourage violence against women.

Violence and Injury

Adolescents are victims of violent crime and theft at twice the rate of adults over 20 years of age (32).

Highlights of AMA policy recommendations on firearms

The AMA encourages and endorses the development and presentation of safety education programs that will engender more responsible use and storage of firearms. The AMA also urges that government agencies—the Centers for Disease Control in particular—enlarge their efforts in the study of firearm-related injuries and in the development of ways and means of reducing such injuries and deaths. The Association urges Congress to enact needed legislation to regulate more effectively the importation and interstate traffic of all handguns, and to support recent legislative efforts to ban the manufacture and importation of nonmetallic, not readily detectable weapons, which resemble toy guns. The AMA encourages the improvement or modification of firearms to make them as safe as humanly possible, and encourages nongovernmental organizations to develop and test new, less hazardous designs for firearms (5).

About 80% of 12-year-olds will be victims of completed or attempted crimes during their lifetimes if current crime rates continue unchanged, and half will be victimized two or more times (32).

Violence and injury account for three fourths of the almost 20,000 adolescent deaths each year (see chapter 1) (49).

Most 10- to 19-year-old homicide victims are killed with guns. In 1987, firearms accounted for 68% of the 1,744 adolescents murdered. Eighteen percent of adolescent homicide victims were murdered with knives and other cutting or stabbing instruments. Fourteen percent were killed with a club or other blunt instrument, killed with personal weapons (hands, fists, etc.), strangled, or murdered by some other means (48).

For every adolescent fatally injured, there are 41 adolescents who are hospitalized and 1,100 who are treated in emergency departments as a result of an injury (101). Additional information on nonfatal injuries appears in question 4 in this chapter.

While at school or on a school bus, 34% of 8th and 10th graders report that someone threatened to hurt them, and 13% report having been attacked (19).

Twelve percent of 8th and 10th graders report that someone raped or tried to rape them outside of school, and 18% report that during the past year someone tried to force them to have sex when they did not want to (19).

In a survey of students in the sixth through ninth grades in Rhode Island, 65% of boys and 57% of girls thought it was acceptable for a man to force a woman to have sex if they had dated for more than 6

Definitions of and cautions about abuse and neglect statistics

There is no single, universally used definition of maltreatment, abuse, and neglect. Statistics on abuse and neglect in this volume come primarily from the 1988 Study of National Incidence and Prevalence of Child Abuse and Neglect (85). In that survey, maltreatment, abuse, and neglect were defined as follows:

Maltreatment: A form of physical, sexual, or emotional abuse or neglect of a child, counted as such by community professionals responsible for child welfare. Also included are other forms of maltreatment such as alcoholism, prostitution, or drug abuse, alleged to affect the child in unspecified ways.

Abuse: *Physical abuse* includes beatings and punishment resulting in injury or impairment such as broken bones, burns, or stopped breathing. *Sexual abuse* includes penile penetration of the child, molestation of genitals, or other sexual acts such as exposure, or fondling breasts or buttocks. *Emotional abuse* includes confinement such as binding arms or legs together or tying the child to an object for punishment, overtly hostile or verbal threats or assault such as threats of beating, or other abuse such as withholding food, shelter, sleep, or other necessities.

Neglect: *Physical neglect* includes failure or delay in ensuring that a minor receives medical care for an injury, illness, or impairment, as well as abandonment, lack of supervision for extended periods of time, expulsion from the home, or driving with the child while intoxicated. *Educational neglect* includes permitting chronic truancy, failing to enroll a child of mandatory school age, and refusing to allow or obtain treatment for a diagnosed learning disorder. *Emotional neglect* includes inadequate nurturing or affection, chronic or extreme spouse abuse in the child's presence, permitting the child to abuse drugs or alcohol, or delay or failure to seek psychological care in cases of severe depression or attempted suicide.

Statistics on neglect and abuse from the 1988 Study of National Incidence and Prevalence of Child Abuse and Neglect (U.S. Department of Health and Human Services) underestimate the actual number of adolescents who are victimized because they include only cases where a demonstrable injury occurred as a result of parental abuse or neglect. Therefore, these statistics exclude cases where a child's health or safety was at risk and cases that involve neglect or abuse by people other than parents or parent substitutes.

months. Fifty-one percent of boys and 41% of girls thought it was acceptable for a man to force a woman to have sex if he spent a lot of money on her (118).

In a national sample of college students, 54% of women reported some form of sexual victimization and 25% of men reported sexually victimizing women (43).

Although adolescents are victims of violence, they are offenders in 24% of all violent crimes leading to an arrest (48).

Forty-nine percent of 8th- and 10th-grade boys and 28% of girls in the 8th and 10th grades report having been in at least one fight during the past year involving physical aggression or a weapon (19).

Forty-one percent of 8th- and 10th-grade boys and 24% of girls report that they could obtain a handgun if they so desired (19).

Abuse and Neglect

Adolescents are more likely to be sexually, physically, and emotionally abused than any other age group of children.

- Approximately 26 of every 1,000 12- to 17-year-olds have been victims of abuse or neglect compared to 16 of every 1,000 children between 6 and 11 years of age, 10 per 1,000 children 3 to 5 years of age, and 6 per 1,000 children under the age of 2 (85).

- In 1986, more than 1 million children and teenagers experienced demonstrable injury or impairment as a result of abuse or neglect (85).

Rates of Abuse and Neglect Experienced by Younger and Older Adolescents

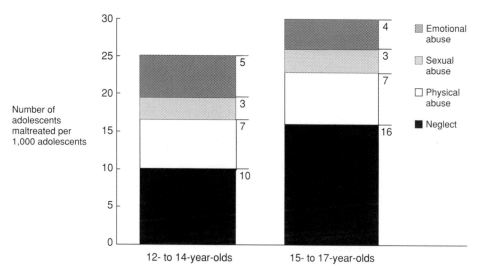

Source: National Center on Child Abuse and Neglect (1988). *Study findings: Study of national incidence and prevalence of child abuse and neglect: 1988* (Contract No. 105-85-1702). Washington, DC: U.S. Department of Health and Human Services.

AMA Profiles of Adolescent Health

◼ Rates of neglect and physical, sexual, and emotional abuse of adolescents appear in the chart (85).

• At least 30 of every 1,000 15- to 17-year-olds and close to 25 of every 1,000 12- to 14-year-olds have been abused or neglected.

• Approximately 56% of maltreated youth were neglected and 48% were abused.

Recurrent or chronic somatic symptoms such as headaches, dizziness, tightness of the chest, loss of appetite, nightmares, insomnia, fear of strangers, unexplained lower abdominal pain (24), and pregnancy or sexually transmitted disease are indicators of possible sexual abuse among early pubertal girls (100, 121).

Abuse or neglect in childhood can have significant implications for mental health and health-compromising behavior during adolescence. There is a strong relationship between previous abuse and depression, suicidal ideation, attempted suicide, sleeping difficulties, and substance abuse during adolescence (6, 50).

2. How prevalent are tobacco, alcohol, and drug use among today's adolescents?

Large numbers of adolescents have tried or currently use tobacco, alcohol, and other drugs. Alcohol and other drugs are factors in many accidents and injuries among adolescents (86). Addiction, poor school performance or dropping out of school, death from accidental drug overdose, and early or unprotected sex are all associated with regular substance use (53). Experimentation with tobacco, alcohol, and other drugs is especially dangerous when it occurs early in adolescence because it can interfere with normal psychosocial development, lead to heavier use,

and disrupt school progress and social relationships with family and friends. Adolescents' attitudes toward tobacco, alcohol, and other drugs are closely tied to whether or not they use them.

There are important differences between adolescents who try a harmful substance once or twice and those who use them more heavily. In the data presented here, the category "ever used" refers to having tried a substance at some time during one's lifetime. Regular or current use of a substance refers to use at least once during the past month. Heavy or "daily" use refers to use at least 20 times or more in the past month.

Limitations of national surveys of substance use

Most data in this chapter come from two prominent national surveys, and both have limitations worth noting. *Monitoring the Future* is a survey of high school seniors funded by the National Institute on Drug Abuse and conducted by the University of Michigan (23, 65, 66). Estimates of substance use from this sample are likely to underestimate actual use among older adolescents. This is because the sample includes only high school seniors, and youth who drop out of school tend to be heavier drug users.

The *NIDA Household Survey on Drug Abuse* interviews members of households in the United States and, therefore, would include high school dropouts (88, 89, 90). However, this survey may also underestimate and skew the picture of substance abuse among adolescents. This is because the survey uses the entire age group of 12- to 17-year-olds as the denominator for calculating the percentage of adolescents who use various substances. For many drugs, such as marijuana and cocaine, however, experimentation begins at about age 15. The inclusion of 12- to 14-year-olds in the denominator "dilutes" the real prominence of substance use among adolescents because relatively few younger adolescents have ever used many drugs. The data on substance use presented in this volume always include either the age or grade level of adolescents in an effort to avoid confusion. (It is worth noting that the NIDA Household Survey also tends to systematically undersample blacks and Hispanics, and for this reason may not accurately represent substance use among these groups.)

Adolescents Who Have Ever Used Tobacco, Alcohol, or Other Drugs

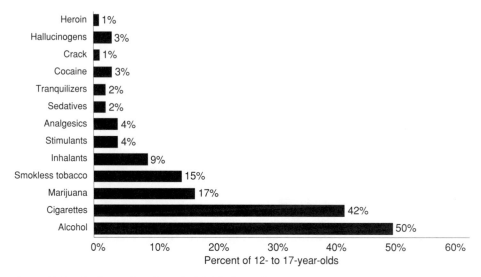

Source: National Institute on Drug Abuse (1989). *Highlights of the 1988 national household survey on drug abuse.* Washington, DC: U.S. Government Printing Office.

AMA Profiles of Adolescent Health

◼ The graph shows the extent to which adolescents have ever used different drugs (90). Three general points should be noted.

• Alcohol and cigarettes are by far the most popular substances tried by 12- to 17-year-olds.

• Marijuana and smokeless tobacco are the next most used substances. About one in six adolescents 12 to 17 years of age has ever used either marijuana or smokeless tobacco.

• Fewer than 10% of adolescents have experimented with most other drugs, but those who do are exposed to serious health risks.

Tobacco Use

More than 8.5 million adolescents between the ages of 12 and 17 (42%) have ever smoked cigarettes (90).

Among 1987 high school seniors:

• 67% reported ever having smoked cigarettes;

• 29% smoked cigarettes within the last month;

• 11% smoked at least 10 cigarettes daily (66).

Since 1977 cigarette smoking has been more common among adolescent girls than boys (115). (Information on trends in cigarette smoking appears in chapter 3, and information on sex differences appears in chapter 4.)

Over 3 million 12- to 17-year-olds (15%) have ever used smokeless tobacco, and 4% are current users. Its use is increasing, especially among young adolescent boys (90).

About 10% of 8th- and 10th-grade boys and 1% of 8th- and 10th-grade girls reported that they currently chew tobacco (19).

Alcohol Use

Although it is illegal to sell alcohol to individuals under 21 years of age, over 10 million 12- to 17-year-olds have ever used alcohol, and many report regular use (90).

In 1988, 50% of 12- to 17-year-olds had tried alcohol at least once, and 6% had consumed it within the past week (89).

Among 1987 high school seniors:

- 92% had consumed alcohol at least once;

- 66% had consumed alcohol within the past 30 days;

- 39% engaged in binge drinking (five or more drinks in a row in the past 2 weeks);

- 5% report daily alcohol use (23).

Drinking and driving is the number 1 killer of adolescents.

- Approximately 12 adolescents between the ages of 15 and 20 are killed each day in alcohol-related accidents (86).

- Close to 20% of all deaths among 15- to 20-year-olds are from alcohol-related car accidents (86).

- Youth under the age of 21 are twice as likely as any other age group to be in an alcohol-related car crash (86).

Marijuana Use

Marijuana is the most widely abused illicit drug among adolescents (90) and is associated with poorer grades, school absenteeism and dropping out of school, rejection of conventional values, low self-esteem, depression, delinquency, and use of other illicit drugs (77).

More than 3.5 million 12- to 17-year-olds (17%) have tried marijuana, and 6% are current users (90).

Among 1987 high school seniors:
- 50% had ever used marijuana;
- 21% were current users;
- 3% were daily users (66).

Consequences of cigarette smoking

Cigarette smoking is linked to cancer, emphysema, and heart disease and is the single most avoidable cause of death in the United States. Smoking accounts for nearly one third of all cancer deaths among adults (19) and can lead to more immediate health problems, such as bronchitis, diminished athletic performance, stained teeth, and bad breath. Research evidence shows that smoking cigarettes at an early age is associated with the use of other drugs (especially for females) and dropping out of high school (77, 122).

Highlights of AMA policy recommendations on tobacco

The AMA supports a tobacco-free society by the year 2000 through the enactment of several policies. The AMA endorses the passage of laws, ordinances, and regulations that would prohibit smoking in public buildings and facilities, prohibit vending machine sales of cigarettes and tobacco products, and set the minimum age for purchasing tobacco products at 21 (13).

The same requirements and restrictions applying to cigarettes should be applied to snuff and chewing tobacco. If there continues to be advertising of snuff and chewing tobacco, the AMA should exert its influence to ensure that there is no exposure of young children and teenagers to the advertising. Also, the AMA urges that manufacturers take steps to diminish the appeal of snuff and chewing tobacco to young persons (44).

The AMA continues to support strong educational efforts, from kindergarten through the 12th grade, to help preteens, adolescents, and young adults avoid the use of tobacco products, including smokeless tobacco. The Association encourages appropriate school authorities to prohibit the use of all tobacco products by students, faculty, and coaches during the school day and during other school-related activities. The AMA encourages the incorporation of appropriate intervention programs with existing educational programs as they are developed (13).

Some youth experiment with marijuana before high school. Fifteen percent of 8th-grade students and 35% of 10th-grade students report that they have used marijuana at least once (19).

Highlights of AMA policy recommendations on illicit drugs

The social, psychological, and medical problems associated with illicit drugs pose major health risks for adolescents. In response to these threats, the AMA has developed recommendations for a comprehensive national policy. The Association calls upon the federal government to recognize that reducing the demand for, as opposed to the supply of, drugs is a realistic approach and that the federal government should take the lead by instituting prevention and intervention programs. To reduce demand, the AMA recommends expanded treatment and rehabilitation programs, a coordinated educational program that complements local educational prevention programs for youth at high risk, a long-term commitment to expanded research and data collection, and recognition of the linkage between drug abuse and use of alcohol and tobacco. The federal government should lead a coordinated approach to adolescent drug education (16).

Shifting the focus away from supply reduction and enforcement does not mean that such efforts should be abandoned. Supply reduction efforts do make importation more difficult, and they symbolize the national commitment to discouraging drug abuse. A shift in emphasis simply means that supply and enforcement programs by themselves are recognized as an inadequate response to drug abuse (16).

Cocaine Use

More than one-half million 12- to 17-year-olds (3%) used cocaine in the past year, and close to one-quarter million are current users (90).

Fifteen percent of 1988 high school seniors reported ever having used cocaine, and more than 3% use it currently (90).

Cocaine (including "crack") use among adolescents places them at high risk for addiction, physical problems, involvement in crime, poor school performance, and dropping out of school.

Use of Other Drugs

The pursuit of physical beauty or athletic prowess has led many adolescents to use nonprescription diet pills or anabolic/androgenic steroids.

• One in six 10th graders (15%) report using nonprescription pills to help control their weight, though only 3% used them on more than 10 occasions (19).

• A recent national survey of high school senior males found that more than 1 in 15 (nearly 7%) had used anabolic/androgenic steroids to enhance either their athletic performance or their appearance (31).

Inhalants are another popular drug among adolescents; almost 10% of 12- to 17-year-olds have sniffed glue (90).

Eleven percent of high school seniors in 1987 had used tranquilizers at least once, and 2% were current users (66).

Eight percent of high school seniors in 1987 had used hallucinogens (e.g., LSD or PCP) at least once, and 2.5% were current users (66).

Overall, 57% of 1987 high school seniors had tried an illicit substance before graduation, and approximately 3% first used an illicit drug in the fifth and sixth grades (66).

HIV infection has been linked to intravenous drug use. Information on HIV and AIDS among adoles-

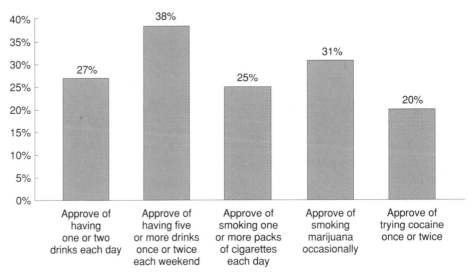

1986 High School Seniors' Approval of Alcohol and Drug Use

Source: Bachman, J. G., Johnston, L. D., & O'Malley, P. M. (1986). *Monitoring the future: Questionnaire responses from the nation's high school seniors, 1986.* Ann Arbor: University of Michigan.

AMA Profiles of Adolescent Health

Highlights of AMA policy recommendations on alcohol

The AMA supports 21 as the legal drinking age, supports strong penalties for providing alcohol to any persons younger than 21 years of age, and supports stronger penalties for providing alcohol to drivers younger than 21 years of age (30). The AMA recommends that producers and distributors of alcoholic beverages discontinue advertising directed toward youth, such as promotions on high school and college campuses. Advertisers and broadcasters should eliminate television program content that depicts the irresponsible use of alcohol without showing its adverse consequences. Examples of such use include driving after drinking, drinking while pregnant, and drinking to enhance performance or win social acceptance (4). The AMA also recommends that health education labels be used on all alcoholic beverage containers and in all alcoholic beverage advertising. The Association urges its constituent state associations to support state legislation to bar the promotion of alcoholic beverage consumption on school (college) campuses and in advertising in school publications (17).

cents appears in question 3 of this chapter and in chapter 3.

■ Adolescents' approval of substance use directly influences the likelihood that they will use them. As the chart shows, significant numbers of 1986 high school seniors approve of heavy use or abuse of alcohol, tobacco, and drugs (23).

- Approximately one in four high school seniors approves of heavy cigarette smoking or having one or two drinks each day.

- Nearly 40% of high school seniors approve of having five or more drinks once or twice each weekend.

- One in five high school seniors approves of trying cocaine.

Many parents are reluctant to believe that drug abuse affects their children. A recent Gallup poll found that 80% of parents of 8- to 17-year-old children thought that drugs were not a problem for their children (52).

Grade of First Use Among 1987 High School Seniors Who Ever Used That Substance

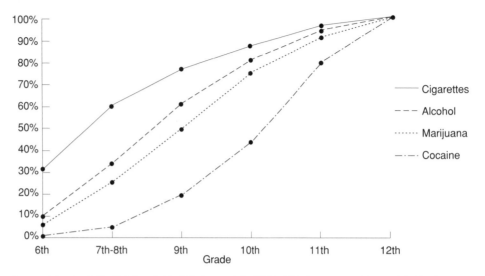

Source: Johnston, L. D., O'Malley, P. M., & Bachman, J. G. (1988). *Illicit drug use, smoking, and drinking by America's high school students, college students, and young adults, 1975-1987* (DHHS Publication No. ADM 89-1602). Washington, DC: U.S. Government Printing Office.

AMA Profiles of Adolescent Health

Age at First Use of Harmful Substances

■ Adolescents begin using different drugs at different ages. As shown in the chart, experimentation with cigarettes and alcohol usually occurs first and experimentation with marijuana and cocaine occurs later. Among the 1987 high school senior class:

• Nearly two of three students who reported having ever used cigarettes first tried them before entering the ninth grade (66).

• One of three students who reported having ever used alcohol first used it before entering the ninth grade (66).

• One of four students who reported having ever used mari-

juana first used it before entering the ninth grade (66).

• One of 20 students who reported having ever used cocaine first used it before entering the ninth grade, and one in five had used it before the 10th grade (66).

Youth who have not experimented with cigarettes, alcohol, or other illicit drugs by the age of 21 are unlikely to do so thereafter (68).

Research shows that use of substances proceeds in stages. Tobacco, alcohol, or marijuana can be "gateway drugs" for adolescents—that is, substances that may lead to the use of other drugs.

Differences Between Adolescent Cigarette Smokers and Nonsmokers in the Use of Other Harmful Substances

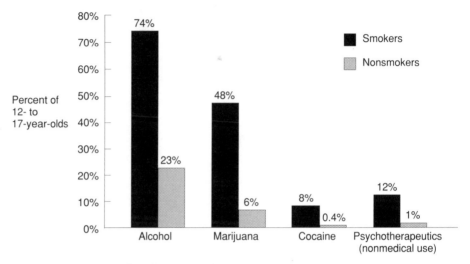

Source: National Institute on Drug Abuse. (1985). *National household survey on drug abuse: Main findings 1985.* Washington, DC: U.S. Government Printing Office.

AMA Profiles of Adolescent Health

The chart above illustrates differences between adolescent cigarette smokers and nonsmokers in the use of other harmful substances (88). Adolescent cigarette smokers are:

- 3 times more likely than nonsmokers to use alcohol currently;

- 8 times more likely to be current users of marijuana;

- 20 times more likely to be current users of cocaine.

Similarly, adolescents who currently drink alcohol are 10 times more likely than nondrinkers to use marijuana and 11 times more likely to use cocaine (88).

Adolescents who currently smoke marijuana are more than 20 times as likely to have tried cocaine than are adolescents who do not smoke marijuana (88).

Adolescents who try alcohol and drugs at an early age are especially likely to continue using drugs throughout adolescence and to use them more heavily (67).

A longitudinal study of adolescents in New York State found that those who were drinking alcohol at age 15 were 30% to 40% more likely to have also used marijuana on more than 10 occasions than were those who started drinking alcohol at age 21 (123).

Of the 6.6% of high school senior males who report having ever used anabolic steroids, 38% used them when they were 15 or younger, and another 35% had started using them by the time they were 16 years old (31).

Ongoing Substance Use

The age at which most adolescents engage in heaviest substance use depends in part on the substance in question.

Regular cigarette smoking increases consistently between the ages of 12 and 18 and remains relatively stable after the age of 18 (68); 35% of 18- to 25-year-olds regularly smoke cigarettes (89).

Use of alcohol peaks at about 19 years of age (before it is legal), when 90% of men and 80% of women are current users. Alcohol use declines sharply after the age of 20 (68).

Marijuana use steadily increases into the early 20s, when 50% of men and 33% of women report current use. Use begins to decline at age 23 (68).

Cocaine use generally begins much later in adolescence or in early adulthood. Use increases after the age of 19 but is generally discontinued by age 28 or 29 (68, 69).

3. How many adolescents are sexually active and how does this threaten their health?

Most people in the United States first experience sexual intercourse during adolescence. Adolescents who engage in early or unprotected sex or who have many partners are especially at risk for unwanted health outcomes.

Initiation of Sexual Activity

A large percentage of American adolescents are sexually active at a young age. By age 16, 29% of boys and 17% of girls have had sexual intercourse. By age 18, these figures increase to 65% for boys and 51% for girls (80).

Highlights of AMA policy recommendations on pregnancy prevention and contraception

The AMA urges print and broadcast media to permit advertising and public service announcements regarding contraception and safer sexual practices as a matter of public health awareness (14). The Association supports responsible sex education that includes accurate and understandable information on sexual responsibility, availability of contraceptives, alternatives in birth control, and other programs aimed at the prevention of teenage pregnancy and sexual transmission of diseases, and emphasizes this stance in its initiative on adolescent health (15). The AMA also believes that premarital sexual abstinence is an effective means of avoiding unwanted pregnancy and other health risks (3).

The AMA continues to oppose regulations that require parental notification when prescription contraceptives are provided to minors through federally funded programs, since they create a breach of confidentiality in the physician-patient relationship (12). The teenage girl whose sexual behavior exposes her to possible conception should have access to medical consultation and the most effective contraceptive advice and methods consistent with her physical and emotional needs. The physician should be free to prescribe or withhold contraceptive advice in accordance with his or her best medical judgment in the best interests of the patient (9). Obstacles to the distribution of birth control information, medication, and devices should be removed and physicians should provide contraceptive services on a confidential basis where legally permissible (10).

A substantial number of sexually active adolescents fail to use contraceptives or use them ineffectively.

- Approximately 50% of American adolescents did not use any contraceptives the first time they had intercourse (59).

- Younger adolescents are less likely than older adolescents to use contraceptives. Forty-two percent of girls under the age of 15 waited a year or more before using contraceptives after they first had sex compared to 35% of 15- to 17-year-olds and 15% of 18- to 19-year-olds (59).

- Of sexually active 15-year-old boys, 36% used no contraceptive or an ineffective method compared to 22% of 17- to 19-year-olds (109).

- Youth are becoming sexually active at a younger age (see chapter 3).

Sexually Transmitted Diseases (STDs)

Sexually transmitted diseases are at epidemic levels among adolescents.

- According to the Centers for Disease Control, 2.5 million adolescents contract a sexually transmitted disease each year (81).

- Fifteen- to 19-year-olds account for approximately 25% of all reported cases of gonorrhea (75).

- About one in four sexually active adolescents will become infected with a sexually transmitted disease before graduating from high school (107).

HIV/AIDS and adolescents

Between 1987 and 1989, less than 0.5% of people with acquired immunodeficiency syndrome (AIDS) were 13 to 19 years of age (36). Sixty-eight percent of adolescents with AIDS contracted it through homosexual or bisexual contact, 13% through intravenous drug use, 8% through homosexual contact and intravenous drug use, 4% through heterosexual contact, 4% from transfusion, and 3% from other sources (120).

Between 1987 and 1989, 20% of people (22,917) with AIDS were 20- to 29-year-olds (35). Because it takes an estimated 5 to 10 years for the human immunodeficiency virus (HIV) infection to result in AIDS, many of these people were adolescents when they became infected with HIV.

Adolescents at highest risk for HIV infection are runaways, youths engaged in prostitution, incarcerated youth, youth with homosexual experience, and intravenous drug users. Adolescents who had first intercourse at an early age and adolescents who have many sexual partners are also at increased risk of HIV infection (120).

Highlights of AMA policy recommendations on HIV/AIDS

The AMA endorses a comprehensive list of recommendations, including the education of elementary, secondary, and college students regarding the modes of HIV transmission and prevention, and the need to work with concerned groups to establish appropriate and uniform policies for youth with HIV disease. The AMA encourages public announcements that include messages on abstinence, condom usage, and safer sex, and encourages specifically targeted messages. Among the audiences that should receive focused messages in an appropriate language and style are intravenous drug users and their sexual partners and minority groups such as blacks and Hispanics. The AMA continues to support a national commission on HIV (18).

The AMA encourages and advocates for an anonymous, representative, cross-sectional study to determine the degree of HIV infection in the United States as a whole, as well as in groups of special interest, such as adolescents and minorities. The study should be repeated at appropriate intervals. The AMA encourages physicians to take a sexual and substance abuse history, sufficient to identify the usual modes of HIV transmission, on every adolescent and adult patient, with a more comprehensive history taken when warranted (18).

- According to one study, homosexual high school students are 23 times more likely than heterosexual students to have had a sexually transmitted disease (99).

- Human papilloma virus (HPV) infections are the most common sexually transmitted disease in the United States and affect as many as 30% of sexually active adolescents in some populations (41).

Like adults, adolescents who have more sexual partners are at greater risk for contracting a sexually transmitted disease.

A national survey of 9th- through 12th-grade students conducted by the Centers for Disease Control found that between 15% and 43% of adolescents (depending on the city they lived in) had three or more sexual partners during their lifetime, thus increasing the chances of contracting a sexually transmitted disease (35).

A Reproductive Profile of Sexually Active Older Adolescent Women

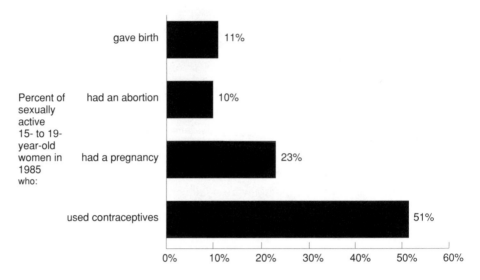

Percent of sexually active 15- to 19-year-old women in 1985 who:

- gave birth — 11%
- had an abortion — 10%
- had a pregnancy — 23%
- used contraceptives — 51%

(x-axis: 0% 10% 20% 30% 40% 50% 60%)

Source: Pittman, K., & Adams, G. (1988). *Teenage pregnancy: An advocate's guide to the numbers.* Washington, DC: Children's Defense Fund.

AMA Profiles of Adolescent Health

Unintended Pregnancy and Early Childbearing

As shown in the chart, the percentage of adolescents who experience pregnancy, abortion, and childbirth reflect the substantial numbers who are sexually active and who fail to use contraceptives or use them ineffectively.

- In 1985, approximately 4.2 million 15- to 19-year-old adolescent women were sexually active (96).

- Among sexually active 15- to 19-year-old women, only half use contraceptives, one in five gets pregnant, 1 in 10 has an abortion, and 1 in 10 gives birth (96).

Most premarital pregnancies are unintended. Approximately 90% of pregnant 15- to 19-year-olds are not married at conception (96).

Of the 472,623 births in 1987 to adolescents younger than 20 years of age, 64% were nonmarital (96).

In 1987 there were 10,311 births to adolescent girls younger than 15 years of age (96).

The Alan Guttmacher Institute estimates that if 1985 rates continue, about 1 in 10 adolescent women (9%) will have given birth by the time they turn 18 (81).

Pregnant adolescents who are in early puberty, who receive late or no prenatal care, who use drugs, who smoke or drink alcohol, and who have a repeat pregnancy within 18 months are especially at risk for poor medical outcomes.

Adolescents who get pregnant while in high school are more likely to drop out of school, become dependent on welfare, and become single parents.

Highlights of AMA policy recommendations on adolescent pregnancy and abortion

The AMA encourages the development of counseling programs that will offer constructive help to expectant mothers in accepting and coping with the stresses of pregnancy, provide emotional support for a decision to continue pregnancy to term, assure availability of adequate information and services regarding adoption in those cases in which the expectant mother might be unable to rear a child, and include educational programs on contraceptive measures appropriate for individual patients (11).

The AMA opposes legislative proposals that utilize federal or state health care funding mechanisms to deny established and accepted medical care to any segment of the population. Abortion is a medical procedure and should be performed only by a duly licensed physician in conformance with standards of good medical practice and the Medical Practice Act of his state. Neither physician, hospital, nor hospital personnel shall be required to perform an act violative of good medical judgment or personally held moral principles. In these circumstances, good medical practice requires only that the physician or other professional withdraw from the case so long as the withdrawal is consistent with good medical practice (3).

4. In what other ways do adolescents' lifestyles place them at risk?

Some adolescents lead dangerous "multiple risk-taking" lifestyles, which means they participate in a constellation of activities that can result in injury, hospitalization, or other unhealthy consequences. Of course, most adolescents do not lead dangerous lives, but neither do they take the precautions they should to ensure good health, such as getting adequate nutrition and exercise.

Multiple Risk-Taking

It has been estimated that 7 million of the 28 million American adolescents between the ages of 10 and 17 are at high risk of poor health outcomes (45).

- These youth engage in many activities that have a high prob-

ability of negative consequences, such as early unprotected sex, abuse of illegal substances, and crime, violence, or delinquency.

- Many of these youth have been held back a year or more in school, have low grades, and are absent from school a great deal; many eventually drop out of school.

- Many of these high-risk youth have already experienced the consequences of high-risk behavior, such as addiction, sexually transmitted diseases, HIV infection, pregnancy, or early parenthood.

Another 7 million youth, one in four, are at moderate risk of poor health outcomes because they engage in some, but not all, of these behaviors (45). These youth experiment with but are not frequent abusers of illegal substances, they are sexually active but use contraceptives, and they do not do well in school but may not yet have failing grades or dropped out.

About half of adolescents are not engaging in behavior that places them at immediate risk for negative health outcomes, but they are exposed to family, school, peer, media, and community influences that could adversely affect their health or behavior (45).

Injuries and Unsafe Behaviors

Due to violence, excessive risk-taking behaviors, or failure to take adequate safety precautions, nonfatal injury rates are higher for adolescents than for any other age group (101).

- Almost half—42 of every 100— of 17- to 24-year-olds are injured each year (66).

- More than half of adolescents (56%) do not use seat belts, and 44% report riding with a driver who has been drinking or using drugs (19).

- Nearly 9 of 10 adolescents ride a bicycle, but 92% never wear a helmet (19).

Of 1986 high school seniors, 35% reported that they get a real kick out of doing things that are a little dangerous, and 45% said that they like to test themselves by doing something a little risky (23).

Nutrition and Exercise

Changes in the American diet, cutbacks in school physical education programs, and relatively inactive lifestyles have contributed to increased obesity and higher cholesterol levels among today's youth.

- Nearly 4 of 10 8th- and 10th-grade students eat fried food four or more times a week (19).

- Of 8th and 10th graders, 45% eat three or more snacks a day, and 61% of these snacks are "junk food," such as soft drinks, candy, doughnuts and other sweets, and ice cream (19).

- Of high school seniors, 40% say that they do not eat breakfast, and fewer than 20% eat fruit or vegetables every day (23).

A national survey of the physical fitness of American youth found that many children and adolescents are in poor physical shape.

- More than half of all girls age 6 to 17 and 25% of boys in the same age group are unable to do a single pull up (i.e., hanging from a bar and pulling the chin to the bar) (97).

- Approximately 50% of girls and 30% of boys 6 to 17 years of age cannot run a mile in less than 10 minutes (98).

Poor performance on cardiorespiratory (heart-lung) endurance tests is related to early fatigue in intellectual and physical activities and can contribute to the development of heart disease later in life (97).

Summary and Implications

Violence and health-damaging behaviors that are part of an overall community or lifestyle cannot be cured within a strictly medical model of health. The solution to these problems requires changes in the knowledge, attitudes, and behavior of adolescents and adults. Available research evidence clearly indicates that the older individuals are when they begin experimenting with tobacco, alcohol, or other drugs, the less likely they are to become regular or heavy users. Similarly, later ages of sexual initiation are also related to more effective contraceptive use and a reduction in unintended pregnancy. It is important to encourage adolescents to avoid or delay risk-taking behavior and to help them find healthy, constructive alternatives.

Chapter

3.

Are adolescents more at risk today than in the past?

Dramatic changes in American society during this century have had profound implications for adolescents' health. Major increases in violence, family disruption, and children growing up in poverty and in single-parent families have created environments that place children at greater risk for health problems as they enter and go through adolescence. New health threats such as the emergence of HIV infection and availability of "crack cocaine" potentially affect all adolescents and make the transition to adulthood more stressful and dangerous than it was for earlier generations.

Despite these grim realities, there have been positive changes in the health of adolescents as well. This chapter reviews the ways in which the health of adolescents has improved and the ways in which it has gotten worse. Whenever data exist, longer-term trends in the health of adolescents are reviewed to see how their health has changed from one generation to another. Recent trends (since 1980) are also described to show short-term changes in the health of today's adolescents.

The questions addressed in this chapter are:

1. In what ways has the health of adolescents improved?

2. In what ways has the health of adolescents gotten worse?

3. What are some of the new threats to adolescents' health?

1. In what ways has the health of adolescents improved?

With the renewed effort to reduce health threats and promote well-being among adolescents, it is easy to forget that certain areas of adolescent health have improved during recent decades. Adolescents today do not need to fear some of the diseases that claimed the lives of earlier generations.

Death

Over the past 50 years, there has been a 67% decline in mortality among 10- to 19-year-olds from 18 per 10,000 to 6 per 10,000 (49).

▰ Trends in death rates among adolescents shown in the graph below (49) indicate the following.

• The death rate due to natural causes fell 90% between 1933 and 1985 but deaths from violence or injury remained fairly stable.

• In 1933 natural causes accounted for more than twice as many deaths as violence or injury, but by 1985 the opposite was true.

Public health efforts and the introduction of vaccines and antibiotics reduced the casualties of polio, measles, pneumonia, and tuberculosis as the major causes of death between 1933 and 1950.

More than 46,000 10- to 19-year-olds alive in 1985 would have died of natural causes just 50 years ago without these dramatic improvements in medical research, practice, and technology.

Chronic Disability

Technological advances in medicine are also primarily responsible for prolonging the lives of children with chronic illness and disabling medical conditions.

Trends in Death Rates Among Adolescents

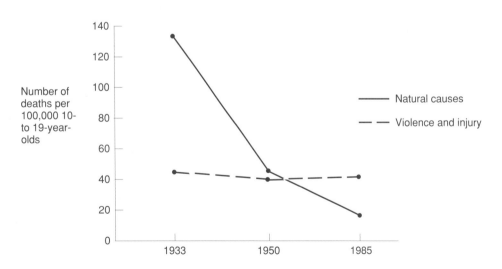

Source: Fingerhut, L. A., & Kleinman, J. C. (1989). *Trends and current status in childhood mortality, United States, 1900-85.* Vital and Health Statistics, Series 3, No. 26 (DHHS Publication No. PHS 89-1410). Hyattsville, MD: National Center for Health Statistics.

- Eighty-four percent of children born with a handicapping condition now survive through the teenage years (55).

- Over 90% of children with severe asthma, juvenile diabetes, sickle cell anemia, and hemophilia will now live at least to 20 years of age (55).

- Over 50% of children with congenital heart disease, cystic fibrosis, and spina bifida will now live to at least 20 years of age (55).

- These figures represent significant improvement in the longevity and quality of life compared to earlier generations.

Healthier Lifestyles

There are recent signs that fewer youth engage in certain unhealthy activities and more youth are beginning to recognize the harmfulness of some activities and take necessary health precautions.

Between 1982 and 1987, there was a 22% drop in alcohol-related traffic fatalities for drivers under the age of 21, an important and encouraging decline because drinking and driving is the number 1 killer of teenagers (86).

Daily cigarette smoking among high school seniors dropped from 29% in 1976 to 19% in 1987 (66).

- The majority of this change, however, occurred between 1978 and 1980 (115).

- The decline in daily cigarette smoking among high school seniors has been greater for males than females, and greater for blacks than whites (see chapter 4, question 6 for details) (115).

Since the late 1970s there has been a decline among 12- to 17-year-olds in the use of marijuana, hallucinogens (such as LSD), sedatives, and tranquilizers (66).

There have been major changes in adolescents' perceptions of the harmfulness of drugs. Between 1975 and 1979, fewer adolescents perceived the use of illicit drugs to be harmful. Since 1979, however, there has been a dramatic increase in the perceived harmfulness of illicit drugs (66).

- The perceived harmfulness of regular marijuana use increased dramatically from 42% in 1979 to 73% in 1987.

- The perceived harmfulness of trying cocaine once or twice also increased considerably from 33% in 1986 to 48% in 1987 (66). It is worrisome that a majority of adolescents do not consider experimentation with cocaine to be harmful.

Condom use at first intercourse reported by males in a national survey almost tripled among 17- to 19-year-olds, from 21% in 1979 to 57% in 1988 (109).

Trends in Rates of Abuse Among Children and Adolescents

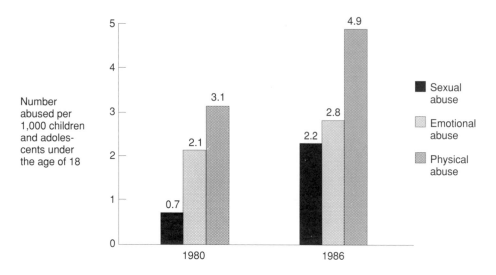

Source: National Center on Child Abuse and Neglect. (1988). *Study findings: Study of national incidence and prevalence of child abuse and neglect: 1988* (Contract No. 105-85-1702). Washington, DC: U.S. Department of Health and Human Services.

AMA Profiles of Adolescent Health

2. In what ways has the health of adolescents gotten worse?

Although improvements in medicine and widespread public health strategies have reduced adolescent mortality as well as cigarette smoking and use of certain drugs, the health of adolescents has gotten worse in several respects.

Death

Suicide and homicide rates increased dramatically during the past 20 years among both younger and older adolescents (49).

- The suicide rate almost tripled among 10- to 14-year-olds between 1968 and 1985 (from 6 to 16 per million) and doubled among 15- to 19-year-olds (from 50 to 100 per million) (49).

- The homicide rate among 10- to 14-year-olds almost doubled between 1968 and 1985 (from 8 to 15 per million). It increased

20% among 15- to 19-year-olds (69 to 86 per million), who already had a significantly higher homicide rate than younger adolescents (49).

Abuse and Neglect

Between 1.0 and 1.5 million children nationwide experienced abuse or neglect in 1986, an alarming 74% increase in reported abuse since 1980 (85).

Although this increase partly reflects improved recognition and reporting of abuse by community professionals, it is cause for great concern. Furthermore, as the graph indicates, there have been increases in all three types of abuse.

- Physical abuse increased 58%, sexual abuse increased 214%, and emotional abuse increased 33% within the past decade (85).

• In 1986, approximately 311,200 youth under the age of 18 were physically abused, 138,000 were sexually abused, and 174,400 were emotionally abused (85).

Mental Health

Many trends in adolescent health (e.g., suicide, drug use) reflect underlying emotional and psychological difficulties. Although the absence of large epidemiological studies make it difficult to detect trends in the prevalence of mental health problems among adolescents, evidence of changes in the utilization of mental health services suggests that more adolescents today are having trouble coping with stresses and problems in their lives, and more have serious psychiatric and psychological problems for which they seek help.

• Between 1966 and 1981, the number of 12- to 17-year-olds who ever received mental health services nearly doubled, from 2% in 1966 to 3.8% in 1981 (126).

• Between 1970 and 1980, the rate of inpatient admissions to psychiatric hospitals increased 10%, from 110 to 121 per 100,000 children under the age of 18 (103).

• In 1986 there were 115,000 youth under the age of 18 who were admitted to a psychiatric hospital. Fifty percent were admitted to a general hospital psychiatric unit, 36% to a private psychiatric hospital, and 13% to a state hospital (91).

The controversy over the psychiatric hospitalization of adolescents

Several diverse factors have contributed to the increased psychiatric hospitalization of adolescents, particularly in private psychiatric hospitals. These factors include a shift away from state and county mental hospitals; divorce or family disruption; decreased stigma of psychiatric treatment; and the availability of insurance policies that reimburse these services rather than less expensive, outpatient services. Critics argue that some parents place their adolescents in hospitals because there is a lack of a continuum of mental health services and because insurance predominantly covers inpatient services (40, 104).

Although the majority of these hospital placements are appropriate, the National Institute of Mental Health (NIMH) estimates that as many as 40% of children and adolescents could have been treated as effectively in an outpatient or residential setting. According to the Congressional Office of Technology Assessment, psychiatric hospital services are often no more effective than nonresidential services provided in the community (91). The factors that contribute to the effectiveness of different psychiatric treatments are complex and will vary depending on the individual patient.

The NIMH and a recent report of the Institute of Medicine estimate that 5 million children and adolescents in the United States need mental health services but do not receive them. Expanding insurance coverage to include partial hospitalization and outpatient visits would help to ameliorate this problem; simply reducing inpatient hospitalization without increasing the availability of a variety of outpatient services would not meet the mental health needs of adolescents.

Estimated Trends in Alcohol and Drug Use Prior to the 10th Grade From the 1950s to the 1980s

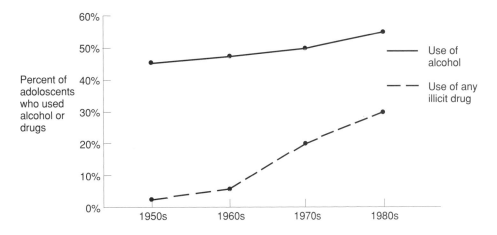

Source: Various sources, in Blane, H. T., & Hewitt, L. E. (1977). *Alcohol and youth: An analysis of the literature, 1960-75* (NIAAA Contract No. ADM-281-75-0026). Springfield, VA: National Technical Information Service. Data for the 1980s are from Johnston, L. D. O'Malley, P. M., & Bachman, J. G. (1988). *Illicit drug use, smoking, and drinking by America's high shcool students, college students, and young adults, 1975-1987* (DHHS Publication No. ADM 89-1602). Washington, DC: U.S. Government Printing Office.

AMA Profiles of Adolescent Health

Substance Use

Although it is difficult to estimate accurately the level of drug or alcohol use by adolescents before 1960, there is evidence that more students are experimenting with drugs at younger ages today, particularly before the 10th grade or age 15.

■ The graph above provides rough estimates of trends in alcohol and drug use before the 10th grade (27). These figures suggest the following.

- During the 1950s, illicit drug use was not widespread among adolescents, particularly before entering high school.

- In the late 1960s and 1970s, however, drug use became more commonplace and more adolescents began experimenting with substances at younger ages.

- By the late 1980s, almost one of every three adolescents had used an illegal substance before entering the 10th grade (66).

- It is estimated that in the 1950s less than half of all adolescents had ever used alcohol before entering high school (27), while in the 1980s, 56% of high school seniors had tried alcohol before they entered the 10th grade (66).

While many types of substance use have declined since the late 1970s, use of certain substances by adolescents has increased. For example, the percentage of high school seniors who had ever used cocaine increased 33% between 1975 and 1988 (from 9% to 12%). Cocaine use among high school seniors peaked in 1985 (at 17%) and has declined recently (66, 90).

Trends in Girls' Sexual Initiation Before Age 16

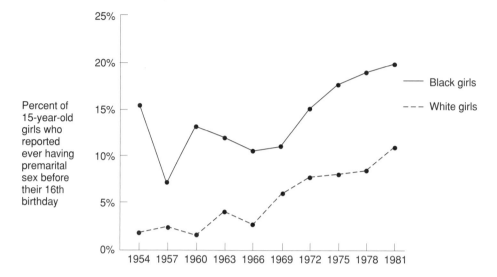

Source: Hofferth, S. L., Kahn, J. R., & Baldwin, W. (1987). Premarital sexual activity among U.S. teenage women over the past three decades. *Family Planning Perspectives, 19,* 46-53.

AMA Profiles of Adolescent Health

Sexual Activity

■ Health risks resulting from sexual activity affect more adolescents today and affect them at younger ages than ever before. The graph above shows trends in girls' sexual initiation by age 16.

• The percentage of white 15-year-old girls who ever had sexual intercourse was 7.5 times greater in 1981 than 1954, having increased from 1.3% to 11%. During the same period, there was a 25% increase among black 15-year-old girls who ever had sexual intercourse, from 16% to 20% (60).

• Historically, black females have been sexually active at younger ages than white females (see chapter 4).

As more adolescents have sexual intercourse, more are contracting sexually transmitted diseases. This is due in part to the delay or failure to use consistently contraceptive measures that are effective in preventing sexually transmitted diseases.

• Cases of reported gonorrhea among 15- to 19-year-old females increased almost 400% in the last 40 years (106).

• Rates of gonorrhea among 10- to 14-year-olds showed a small but steady increase during the same time period (106).

Since the 1950s, adolescents have had sexual intercourse at younger ages, but it is difficult to determine exact long-term effects of this trend on pregnancy, abortion, and birth rates because data in these areas have been available only since 1972.

Trends in Rates of Pregnancy, Abortion, and Births Among Older Adolescent Women

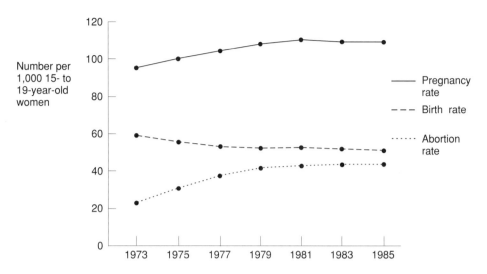

Source: Henshaw, S. K., Kenney, A. M., Somberg, D., & Van Vort, J. (1989). *Teenage pregnancy in the United States: The scope of the problem and state responses.* New York: Alan Guttmacher Institute. © Alan Guttmacher Institute.

AMA Profiles of Adolescent Health

▨ Recent trends in rates of pregnancy, abortion, and births among older adolescent women (shown above) indicate the following.

- The proportion of 15- to 19-year-olds who became pregnant increased during the 1970s but has remained steady since then, with about 11% becoming pregnant each year (57).

- Following the legalization of abortion, the rate of abortion increased during the 1970s but has remained fairly steady since then, with just over 4% of 15- to 19-year-olds having abortions each year (57).

- The birth rate among 15- to 19-year-olds declined slightly during the 1970s and has been steady during the 1980s at about 55 births per 1,000 women (57).

Pregnancy, abortion, and birth rates among adolescents younger than 15 are much lower than those of 15- to 19-year-olds, but trends through time are similar (81). Between 1973 and 1987:

- The pregnancy rate for adolescents younger than 15 increased 23%, from 13.5 to 16.6 per 1,000 (57).

- The abortion rate increased 62%, from 5.6 to 9.1 per 1,000 (57).

- The birth rate declined by 10%, from 6.1 to 5.5 per 1,000 (57).

Trends in Race Differences in Nonmarital Births Among Older Adolescents

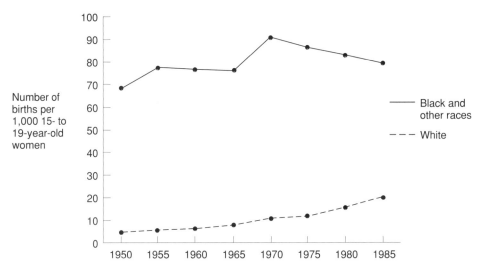

Source: U.S. Department of Education. (1988). *Youth indicators, 1988: Trends in the well-being of American youth.* Washington, DC: U.S. Government Printing Office.

AMA Profiles of Adolescent Health

■ The graph above shows that nonmarital births among adolescents increased between the 1950s and the 1980s, especially among white women under 20 years of age.

• Nonmarital births among white adolescents increased 300%, from 5.1 per 1,000 in 1950 to 20.5 per 1,000 in 1985 (113).

• Nonmarital births among black adolescents increased 16%, from 68.5 per 1,000 in 1950 to 79.4 per 1,000 in 1985, having peaked in 1970 at 90.8 births per 1,000 (113).

As recently as 1970, only 30% of births to women under age 20 were nonmarital. By 1987 two thirds (64%) of all births to adolescents under 20 years of age were nonmarital (81).

Despite year-to-year fluctuations, rates of violence, abuse, sexually transmitted diseases, nonmarital births, and use of alcohol, smokeless tobacco, and some other drugs have increased during the past 20 years among adolescents and affected them at younger ages.

3. What are some of the new threats to adolescents' health?

Although many of the negative trends noted above are disturbing, there are new health threats that deserve special attention. These include the lethal human immunodeficiency virus (HIV), which

causes the acquired immunodeficiency syndrome (AIDS), the widespread availability of cocaine and "crack," and the use of anabolic/androgenic steroids.

HIV and AIDS

The actual rate of HIV infection among adolescents is not known. However, recent studies have found that 1 of 1,000 17- to 19-year-old military recruits and 2 of 1,000 college students were infected with HIV (34, 73).

Because it can take several years for someone infected with HIV to develop AIDS (37), adolescents diagnosed today with HIV will probably be in their 20s before they develop AIDS.

Approximately 23,000 people diagnosed with AIDS are between 20 and 29 years of age. They represent 20% of people currently diagnosed as having AIDS (36).

About 440 adolescents 13 to 19 years of age were diagnosed as having AIDS between 1981 and 1989, which represents fewer than 1% of all AIDS cases (36).

Cocaine

Cocaine and its newer derivatives, such as crack, are highly addictive and have infiltrated the lives of adolescents as well as adults.

Between 1972 and 1988, cocaine use (within the last 12 months) among 12- to 17-year-olds almost doubled, from 1.5% to 2.9%. Cocaine use in this age group peaked between 1979 and 1985, when 4% had used it in the preceding year (90).

Use of cocaine in the preceding year among 18- to 25-year-olds increased 50%, from 8% in 1974 to 12% in 1985 (90).

Between 1984 and 1986, the pro-portion of high school seniors who said they had ever used cocaine, and could not stop when they tried, doubled from 0.4% to 0.8% (65).

There is growing concern over the health consequences of increased participation in prostitution, theft, and other criminal activities to support cocaine addiction.

• The combination of prostitution and intravenous drug use can result in sexually transmitted disease, HIV infection, and giving birth to cocaine-dependent and developmentally disabled babies.

• Drug-related criminal activities expose youth to homicide, violence, and nonfatal injury.

Anabolic/Androgenic Steroids

There is growing concern about increased use of anabolic/andro-genic steroids among adolescents, though there is very little information about the numbers and characteristics of youth who use them.

Steroid use is thought to be more prevalent among boys than girls and higher among athletes than nonathletes. It is estimated that as many as 6.6% of high school males (31) and 2.5% of high school females use or have used anabolic steroids (111).

While not all of the health consequences associated with steroid use are known, their use by adolescents is particularly distressing because they can result in premature closure of the epiphyses (i.e., the two growing ends of the long bones of the arms and legs) or decreased hormone production, which can, in turn, decrease fertility (31).

Summary and Implications

Advances in medical research, practice, and technology have dramatically reduced deaths due to natural causes and substantially prolonged the lives of chronically ill adolescents. However, these gains have been partially offset by increases in violent death and injury. There are hopeful signs of decreased substance abuse among adolescents, though abuse levels remain far too high.

Medical approaches alone cannot prevent or diminish many of the major contemporary threats to adolescent health from violence, abuse and neglect, use of tobacco, alcohol, and drugs, unsafe sexual practices, and psychological problems. To reverse the trend in which serious health threats affect more adolescents at younger ages, we must actively promote healthy behavior by strengthening families, schools, and communities, and creating healthier environments for today's youth. Highlights of health-promoting efforts for adolescents conducted by government, business, private foundations, organized medicine, and communities appear in chapter 5.

4.

Which adolescents are more at risk for particular health problems?

There is a tendency to think of adolescents as a homogeneous group. Although many health threats potentially affect all adolescents, some adolescents are more at risk than others because of their behavior, environment, or personal and family characteristics. It is important to understand the degree to which different groups are vulnerable to specific health threats in order to target effective prevention and intervention strategies. This chapter examines the prevalence of various health problems among different groups of adolescents, depending on their age, sex, family income, race or ethnicity, and sexual orientation.

Many people have misconceptions about how vulnerable different groups are to various health threats. For example, drug abuse is considered by many to be a problem primarily for inner city, minority youth. However, available data show that the problem is far more widespread. The purpose of this chapter is to correct such misconceptions and gauge the degree to which different groups of adolescents are affected by particular health threats.

The questions addressed in this chapter are:

1. **Which adolescents are more likely to die?**

2. **Which adolescents are more likely to experience abuse?**

3. **Which adolescents are more at risk for mental disorders?**

4. **Which adolescents are more likely to be injured?**

5. **Which adolescents are less likely to get the health care they need?**

6. Which adolescents are more likely to use alcohol, tobacco, or drugs?

7. Which adolescents are more likely to get pregnant, have abortions, give birth, or contract a sexually transmitted disease?

8. How do differences in age at first intercourse, sexual activity, and contraceptive use affect the likelihood of getting pregnant or contracting a sexually transmitted disease?

1. Which adolescents are more likely to die?

There are important differences in death rates among different age and race groups and between males and females. Because U.S. death certificates do not include information about family income, it is difficult to determine the effects of poverty on causes and rates of mortality, independent of race. However, because 3 times as many black children as white children

under age 18 live in poverty, racial differences in death rates probably reflect socioeconomic differences as well (49).

Age Differences

The overall death rate is 3 times greater for older than younger adolescents due primarily to differences in motor vehicle deaths, homicide, and suicide (49).

Differences in Leading Causes of Death Between Younger and Older Adolescents

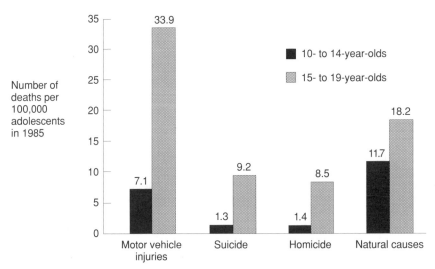

Source: Fingerhut, L. A., & Kleinman, J. C. (1989). *Trends and current status in childhood mortality, United States, 1900-85*. Vital and Health Statistics, Series 3, No. 26 (DHHS Publication No. PHS 89-1410). Hyattsville, MD: National Center for Health Statistics.

Differences in Leading Causes of Death Between Black and White Adolescents

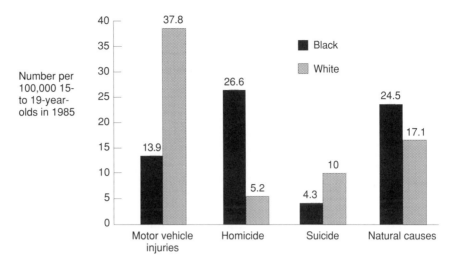

Source: Fingerhut, L. A., & Kleinman, J. C. (1989). *Trends and current status in childhood mortality, United States, 1900-85.* Vital and Health Statistics, Series 3, No. 26 (DHHS Publication No. PHS 89-1410). Hyattsville, MD: National Center for Health Statistics.

AMA Profiles of Adolescent Health

■ Differences in leading causes of death between younger and older adolescents appear in the graph on page 48.

• Motor vehicle death rates are nearly 5 times greater for 15- to 19-year-olds than 10- to 14-year-olds, suicide deaths are 7 times greater, and homicide deaths are 6 times greater (49).

• Death rates from the leading natural causes are 1.5 times greater among 15- to 19-year-olds than 10- to 14-year-olds (49).

Sex Differences

Among 15- to 19-year-olds, males are 4 times more likely than females to die of suicide, 3 times more likely to die of homicide, and 2.5 times more likely to die of motor vehicle injuries (49).

Adolescent girls are 5 times more likely than boys to attempt suicide, but adolescent boys are 4 times more likely actually to commit suicide (28).

Among 10- to 14-year-olds, boys are 4 times more likely than girls to die of drowning (49).

Race and Ethnic Differences

■ Although the death rate for *older* black and white youth is the same—81 deaths per 100,000—there are striking differences in causes of death (49), indicated in the graph above.

• Whites between the ages of 15 and 19 are nearly 3 times more likely than blacks to die of motor vehicle injuries and twice as likely to die of suicide (49).

• Black 15- to 19-year-olds, however, are 5 times more likely than whites to die of homicide, 2 times more likely to die of drowning, and 1.4 times more likely to die of natural causes (49).

Among *younger* adolescents, the overall death rate is 27% greater among blacks than whites (49). Ten- to 14-year-old black adolescents are:

• 4 times more likely than whites to die of drowning;

• 3 times more likely to die of homicide or fire;

• only half as likely to die of suicide (49).

The death rate among Native American and Alaskan native 15- to 24-year-olds is 1.7 times greater than among whites of the same ages (114).

• The suicide rate among 10- to 14-year-old Native Americans and Alaskan natives is 4.6 times greater than among all other groups (6.9 and 1.5 per 100,000, respectively). Among 15- to 19-year-olds, the suicide rate is 2.6 times greater than for other groups (26.3 vs. 10.2 per 100,000, respectively) (112).

Asian American adolescents experience the lowest rates of unintentional injury deaths (approximately half the rate of whites). Suicide and homicide rates among Asian Americans are also lower than among whites. However, there may be wide variation in injury deaths among Asian American subgroups (25).

Differences in Physical, Sexual, and Emotional Abuse of Children and Adolescents

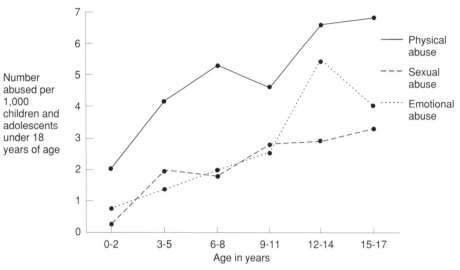

Source: National Center on Child Abuse and Neglect. (1988). *Study findings: Study of national incidence and prevalence of child abuse and neglect: 1988* (Contract No. 105-85-1702). Washington, DC: U.S. Department of Health and Human Services.

AMA Profiles of Adolescent Health

2. Which adolescents are more likely to experience abuse?

Although abuse can and does affect all types of children in all types of families, it is more common among females and youth from low-income family backgrounds. Research evidence is mixed on race differences in sexual abuse. National data on ethnic differences in abuse are not available.

Age Differences

■ Age differences in physical, sexual, and emotional abuse from childhood through adolescence are illustrated in the graph above.

• Between childhood and early adolescence, rates of physical abuse increase by 45% and emotional abuse increases by 100% (85).

• While rates of sexual and physical abuse are slightly higher among 15- to 17-year-olds than

among younger adolescents, rates of emotional abuse are lower (85).

Sex Differences

Although the rates of physical and emotional abuse are very similar for males and females, rates of sexual abuse are 4 times greater among females (85).

Race and Ethnic Differences

A 1986 survey of community professionals in state Child Protective Services agencies, schools, hospitals, and police departments did not find significant race differences in any type of abuse or neglect (85).

However, a 1987 national household survey found race differences in sexual abuse. Thirteen percent of white females and 8% of black

Differences in Reported Abuse Rates by Family Income

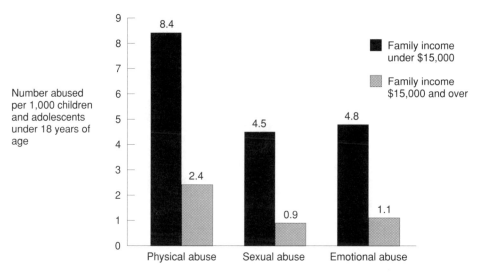

Source: National Center on Child Abuse and Neglect. (1988). *Study findings: Study of national incidence and prevalence of child abuse and neglect: 1988* (Contract No. 105-85-1702). Washington, DC: U.S. Department of Health and Human Services.

AMA Profiles of Adolescent Health

females said that they were forced to have sex at least once before age 20. Six percent of black males and 2% of white males also reported nonvoluntary sex (82).

Inconsistent findings between these studies on race differences in sexual abuse may reflect differences between household reporting and social service agency records. Individuals in households may report abuse of which social service agencies are not aware.

Family Income Differences

■ Family income has a profound effect on reported rates of abuse and neglect. As seen in the graph above, children and adolescents in low-income families are:

- 3.5 times more likely to be physically abused;

- 5 times more likely to be sexually abused;

- over 4 times more likely to be emotionally abused (85).

Poor children are also more than 8 times more likely to suffer serious injury or impairment because of abuse (85).

Surveys of child welfare authorities may underestimate the amount of abuse experienced by adolescents in middle- and upper-income families because their parents may be able to avoid having maltreatment reported to authorities.

3. Which adolescents are more at risk for mental disorders?

Youth with a mental disorder or who experience psychological distress are more likely than other youth to engage in behavior that endangers their health. In order to develop effective prevention and intervention programs for at-risk

Mental health problems of gay and lesbian youth

The Report of the Secretary's Task Force on Youth Suicide indicated that "gay and lesbian youth face extreme physical and verbal abuse, rejection and isolation from family and peers. They often feel totally alone and socially withdrawn out of fear of adverse consequences. As a result of these pressures, lesbian and gay youth are more vulnerable than other youth to psychosocial problems including substance abuse, chronic depression, school failure, early relationship conflicts, being forced to leave their families, and having to survive on their own prematurely. Each of these problems presents a risk factor for suicidal feelings and behavior among gay, lesbian, bisexual, and transsexual youth." Two thirds of gay and bisexual boys report serious substance abuse problems, including chemical dependency (54).

groups of adolescents, it is important to know which youth are most at risk of developing a mental disorder, depending on their family background, social environment, and other factors.

According to the Institute of Medicine (63), youth at high risk of developing a mental disorder include those who:

- have parents who are mentally ill or who abuse alcohol or other substances;

- experience prolonged separation from parents;

- lack continuity of caretakers;

- live with parents in discordant marriages or in unstable families;

- live in foster care;

- have a chronic medical illness;

- live in crowded inner-city neighborhoods;

- live in poverty;

- are homeless;

- have been physically neglected or abused;

- have experienced catastrophic events or bereavement;

- are Native American children from certain tribes whose risk of suicide may be more than double the rate for the U.S. population of the same age group.

Socioeconomic differences have a more pronounced impact than age, race, or sex on the risk of mental illness and disability among adolescents.

4. Which adolescents are more likely to be injured?

It is difficult to estimate injury rates for adolescents because available national data exist only for either the 5- to 17-year-old age group or all youth under the age of 18 years. This limitation may conceal important differences among children, young adolescents, and older adolescents. Nonetheless, there are important sex, race, and income differences in injury rates.

Sex Differences

The nonfatal injury rate for children between the ages of 5 and 17 is almost 30% greater for boys than girls (33.6 and 26 per 100 persons, respectively) (1).

Race and Ethnic Differences

The nonfatal injury rate for children under the age of 18 is 70%

greater among whites than blacks (31 and 18 per 100 persons, respectively) (1).

Family Income Differences

Although the injury rate is the same for the poor and nonpoor

(about 16 injuries per 1,000 among 5- to 17-year-olds), children and adolescents in poverty seem to suffer more serious injuries. They have twice as many restricted activity days (1).

5. Which adolescents are less likely to get the health care they need?

It is difficult to get a clear picture of health care utilization or the prevalence of various medical conditions among adolescents. Most national data on these topics combine children and adolescents into age groups that are under 18 years of age or 5 to 17 years of age. Data on racial and ethnic minorities are generally restricted to white and black comparisons, although there are probably differences in health care utilization among cultural subgroups of both Hispanic and Asian American adolescents.

Sex Differences

Almost three-fourths of both boys and girls 12 to 17 years of age had contact with a physician during the past year, and 3.5% were hospitalized (excluding obstetrical deliveries) (1).

While about 55% of both boys and girls 5 to 17 years of age received medical attention for an acute medical condition in 1988 (1), girls were more likely than boys to:

• have an acute condition;

• spend more days in bed because of health reasons;

• miss more days of school because of an acute medical condition.

In a survey of 8th and 10th graders, girls were twice as likely as

boys to report finding it very hard to cope with stresses at home and school, to often feel sad and hopeless, and to have nothing to look forward to during the preceding month (see chapter 1, question 3) (19).

Race and Ethnic Differences

White children under 18 years of age are more likely than black children to:

• have a reported acute medical condition;

• have more days of limited activities due to poor health;

• spend more days in bed because of health reasons;

• miss more days of school for health reasons (1).

Among 12- to 14-year-olds, whites are slightly more likely than blacks to have been hospitalized during the past year (2.3% and 1.7%, respectively). Among 15- to 17-year-olds, however, 3.5% of both blacks and whites have had a hospital visit (excluding obstetrical deliveries) (1).

More Native Americans under 15 years of age were hospitalized than were non-Native Americans (608 and 513 discharges per 10,000 children, respectively) (76).

Differences in Health Status of Children and Adolescents by Family Income

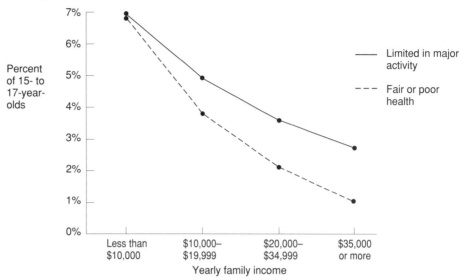

Source: Adams, P. F., & Hardy, A. M. (1989). *Current estimates from the national health interview survey, 1988.* Vital and Health Statistics, Series 10, No. 173 (DHHS Publication No. 89-1501). Hyattsville, MD: National Center for Health Statistics.

AMA Profiles of Adolescent Health

Family Income Differences

Children and adolescents in poverty have 1.7 times more short-term hospital stays and 1.4 times more disability days in which they miss school than youth in families with annual incomes over $35,000 (1).

■ Other differences in the health status of children and adolescents as a function of family income appear in the graph above.

• Children in poverty are nearly 7 times more likely than children in families with annual incomes over $35,000 to be in fair or poor health (1).

• Children in poverty are 2.5 times more likely to be limited in a major daily activity (such as school attendance) because of a chronic condition (1).

Differences in Current Substance Use Between Adolescents and Young Adults

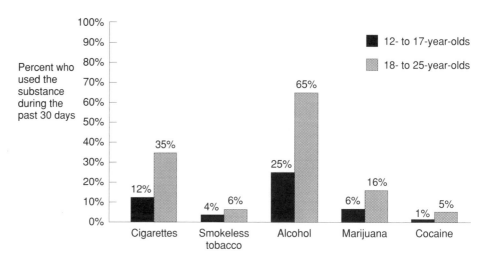

Source: National Institute on Drug Abuse. (1989). *National household survey on drug abuse: Population estimates 1988* (DHHS Publication No. ADM 89-1636). Washington, DC: U.S. Government Printing Office.

AMA Profiles of Adolescent Health

6. Which adolescents are more likely to use alcohol, tobacco, or drugs?

Television and newspapers often portray drug use as a problem primarily of high-school-age students and minorities. According to some surveys, however, adolescent substance use often starts among younger students (see chapter 2, question 2) and is more prevalent among young adults and among whites.

Age Differences

Although drug use is often considered an adolescent problem, the graph shows that current use of many substances is actually more prevalent among young adults 18 to 25 years of age.

Drug use is greater in large urban areas

Twelve- to 17-year-olds living in large cities are 1.5 times more likely to try cocaine and 1.3 times more likely to try marijuana than adolescents in nonmetropolitan areas (88).

- Current use of cigarettes and marijuana is almost 3 times greater among young adults, alcohol use is 2.6 times greater, cocaine use is 5 times greater, and use of smokeless tobacco is 1.5 times greater (89).

Young adults are also heavier users than adolescents. For example, 4% of 12- to 17-year-olds and 10% of 18- to 25-year-olds who ever used marijuana use it once a week or more (89).

Sex Differences

In general, 12- to 17-year-old boys and girls are equally likely to have tried alcohol and other drugs, but boys are:

- twice as likely as girls to be heavy drinkers;

- 7 times more likely ever to have used smokeless tobacco (89).

Race and Ethnic Differences Among Adolescents Who Ever Used Cigarettes, Alcohol, or Other Drugs

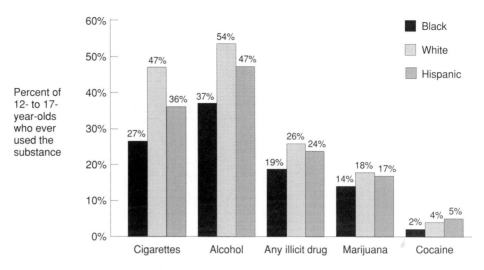

Source: National Institute on Drug Abuse. (1989). *National household survey on drug abuse: Population estimates 1988* (DHHS Publication No. ADM 89-1636). Washington, DC: U.S. Government Printing Office.

AMA Profiles of Adolescent Health

Since 1977, daily cigarette smoking has been consistently greater among female than male high school seniors. In 1987, 20% of female and 16% of male high school seniors smoked cigarettes daily (115).

Race and Ethnic Differences

It is difficult to assess differences in drug use among racial and ethnic groups because of limitations in data sources. Surveys of drug use generally underestimate minority drug use due to sampling or data collection procedures. The best evidence available suggests that drug use is more prevalent among whites than other groups.

■ White 12- to 17-year-olds are more likely than minority youth to experiment with alcohol, tobacco, and most other drugs (89). The chart above shows the following

race and ethnic differences for 12- to 17-year-olds.

• Whites are 1.7 times more likely than blacks and 30% more likely than Hispanics ever to have used cigarettes.

• Whites are 1.5 times more likely than blacks and 15% more likely than Hispanics ever to have used alcohol.

• Whites are 1.4 times more likely than blacks to have tried an illicit drug.

• Whites are 1.3 times more likely than blacks ever to have used marijuana.

Hispanic adolescents are more likely than either black or white adolescents ever to have used cocaine (89).

Native American adolescents are more likely than whites ever to

Race and Ethnic Differences in Heavy Substance Use* Among Adolescents Who Ever Used That Substance

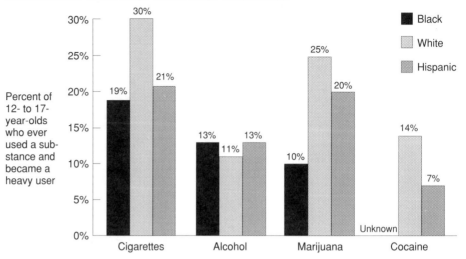

* Heavy use is defined as once a week or more except for cigarette use, where it is use in the past month.

Source: National Institute on Drug Abuse. (1989). *National household survey on drug abuse: Population estimates 1988* (DHHS Publication No. ADM 89-1636). Washington, DC: U.S. Government Printing Office.

AMA Profiles of Adolescent Health

have used alcohol, marijuana, cocaine, and various other substances, though the size of the difference varies among surveys and tribes (112).

Native American adolescents begin abusing various substances at younger ages than do other racial and ethnic groups and are more likely to use multiple drugs in combination (112).

White 12- to 17-year-olds are more likely than black or Hispanic youth to be heavy users of all harmful substances except alcohol (89).

◼ Shown in the graph are racial and ethnic differences in the percentages of youth who ever tried a substance and subsequently became a heavy user.

- Slightly more than 1 in 10 black, white, and Hispanic adolescents who ever used alcohol subsequently became heavy users (89).

- Nearly one in three whites who ever used cigarettes subsequently smoked regularly, compared to only one in five Hispanics or blacks (89).

Differences in drug use among Hispanic subgroups

Data for Hispanics often conceal important subcultural differences in prevalence of use and preference for different substances. A recent report (87) on drug use among Mexican American, Puerto Rican, and Cuban American adolescents found the following.

• Mexican Americans were 20% *more* likely than Puerto Ricans and 50% more likely than Cubans ever to have used marijuana.

• Mexican Americans were 70% *less* likely than Puerto Ricans and only 33% as likely as Cubans ever to have tried cocaine.

The age range used in the survey was 12 to 24 years of age for Cubans and 12 to 17 years of age for Mexican Americans and Puerto Ricans. Thus, the comparison of cocaine use between Mexican American and Cuban American adolescents may be a function of age differences.

- About one in four white adolescents who ever used marijuana subsequently became heavy users, compared to one in five Hispanics and 1 in 10 blacks (89).

- About one in eight white adolescents who ever used cocaine subsequently became heavy users, compared to 1 in 16 Hispanics (data for blacks were not reported because of low statistical reliability) (89).

In the overall U.S. population, blacks are more likely than whites to smoke cigarettes on a daily basis. However, among 1987 high school seniors, daily cigarette smoking was less common among blacks (8%) than whites (20%) (115). These differences reflect, in part, the positive effect of educational attainment on smoking and differences between the dropout rates of blacks and whites.

7. Which adolescents are more likely to get pregnant, have abortions, give birth, or contract a sexually transmitted disease?

Age and race are strongly related to the likelihood of adolescent pregnancy, abortion, and sexually transmitted disease. Adolescents who give birth before they reach 20 years of age are more likely to drop out of school and become dependent on welfare than their peers who do not experience early childbearing. In general, poor and minority adolescents are more at risk than other youth for pregnancy, abortion, or sexually transmitted disease. Other factors that influence these outcomes are discussed in question 8.

Age Differences

In 1985, 3% of adolescent pregnancies were in girls under the age of 15, 36% were in women 15 to 17 years old, and 61% were in women 18 to 19 years old (96).

Over 90% of adolescents under the age of 15 who gave birth in 1985 were unmarried, compared to 71% of 15- to 17-year-olds and 51% of 18- to 19-year-olds (96).

In 1985, over half (54%) of pregnancies among adolescents younger than 15 ended in abortion, compared to 42% of pregnancies among 18- to 19-year-olds (96).

Gonorrhea rates are higher among sexually active 15- to 19-year-olds than 20- to 24-year-olds (21).

Race and Ethnic Differences in Pregnancy, Abortion, and Birth Rates Among Older Adolescent Women

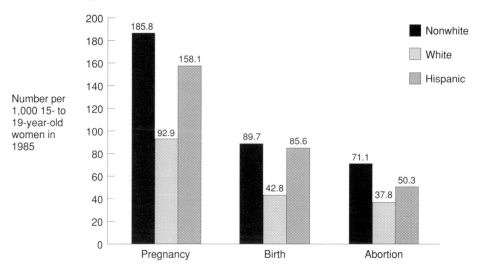

Source: Henshaw, S. K., Kenney, A. M., Somberg, D., & Van Vort, J. (1989). *Teenage pregnancy in the United States: The scope of the problem and state responses.* New York: Alan Guttmacher Institute. © The Alan Guttmacher Institute.

AMA Profiles of Adolescent Health

Race and Ethnic Differences

▬ Major race and ethnic differences exist in pregnancy, abortion, and birth rates among older adolescent women, indicated in the chart.

- The pregnancy rate is 2 times greater for blacks than whites and 1.7 times greater for Hispanics than whites (57).

Shortcomings of national fertility data

National data on racial and ethnic *trends* in pregnancy, abortion, and marital and nonmarital births do not exist except for black and white Americans. This is because past surveys categorized Hispanics, Asians, and Native Americans as "white," or grouped them together with blacks in a "nonwhite" category.

- The abortion rate is almost 1.9 times greater for blacks than whites and 1.3 times greater for Hispanics than whites (57).

- The birth rate for blacks and Hispanics is more than two times the birth rate for whites (57).

In 1985, only 5% of Asian births were to adolescents compared with 20% of all nonwhite births. Asians accounted for only 1% of births to all mothers younger than 15 (61).

In 1985, black adolescent girls were 4 times more likely than whites to have a nonmarital birth (96). (See chapter 3, question 2 for trends in race differences in nonmarital births.)

About 42% of both whites and nonwhites end their pregnancies in abortion (57).

Race Differences in Gonorrhea Rates Among Older Adolescent Women

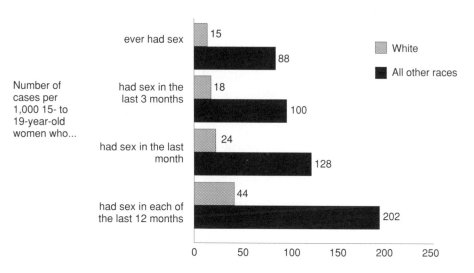

Source: 1982 data, in Aral, S. O., Schaffer, J. E., Mosher, W. D., & Cates, W., Jr. (1988). Gonorrhea rates: What denominator is most appropriate? *American Journal of Public Health, 78,* 702-703.

AMA Profiles of Adolescent Health

Gonorrhea rates are more than 7 times greater among nonwhite 15- to 19-year-old women than white women (50 vs. 7 cases per 1,000 women, respectively) (21).

As shown in the chart, gonorrhea rates among sexually active black 15- to 19-year-olds are 5 to 6 times greater than among whites, regardless of level of sexual activity (21).

Race and Ethnic Differences in the Percentage of Sexually Active Adolescent Men

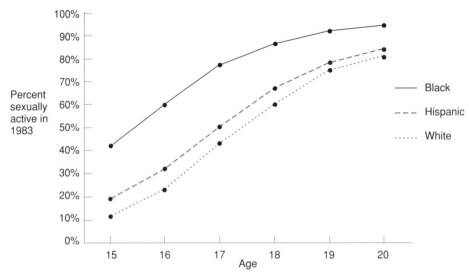

Source: National Longitudinal Survey of Youth, 1983, in Hofferth, S. L., & Hayes, C. D. (Eds.). (1987). *Risking the future: Adolescent sexuality, pregnancy, and childbearing* (Vol. 1). Washington, DC: National Academy Press.

AMA Profiles of Adolescent Health

8. How do differences in age at first intercourse, sexual activity, and contraceptive use affect the likelihood of getting pregnant or contracting a sexually transmitted disease?

Racial and ethnic differences in age at first intercourse, and the effective and consistent use of contraceptives, partially explain differences in pregnancy rates and rates of sexually transmitted disease.

◼ As shown in the graphs above and on the following page, blacks are much more likely than whites to be sexually active at younger ages, regardless of sex (58).

• Regardless of age, black adolescent males and females are more likely to have had sexual intercourse than either whites or Hispanics (58).

• By age 15, black males are 3.5 times more likely than white males, and twice as likely as Hispanic males, to have had intercourse (58).

• By age 15, black females are twice as likely as white females, and 2.5 times as likely as Hispanic females, to have had intercourse (58).

• Regardless of age, Hispanic males are *more* likely than white males to be sexually active. However, Hispanic female adolescents are *equally or less* likely than white females to be sexually active regardless of age (58).

• By age 15, boys are more than twice as likely as girls of the same race or ethnicity to have had sexual intercourse. By age 19, they are only 1.2 times as likely to have had sexual intercourse (58).

It is estimated that 20% of all premarital adolescent pregnancies occur within the first month of

Race and Ethnic Differences in the Percentage of Sexually Active Adolescent Women

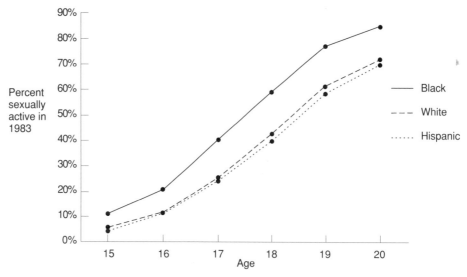

Source: National Longitudinal Survey of Youth, 1983, in Hofferth, S. L., & Hayes, C. D. (Eds.). (1987). *Risking the future: Adolescent sexuality, pregnancy, and childbearing* (Vol. 1). Washington, DC: National Academy Press.

AMA Profiles of Adolescent Health

having sexual intercourse for the first time, and half occur within 6 months of first intercourse (124).

Delay and inconsistent use of contraceptives is much more common among adolescents who have first intercourse before age 15 (59).

• Of adolescent girls under the age of 15, 42% delay contraceptive use by more than 12 months after first intercourse, compared to 35% of 15- to 17-year-olds and only 15% of 18- to 19-year-old women (59).

• A 1988 national survey found that more than 60% of 15- to 19-year-old sexually active men used a condom at first intercourse, compared with 48% of those who had intercourse between the ages of 12 and 14 (109).

Contraceptive use increases with age for both white and black fe-

males, but blacks are much more likely to delay contraceptive use for more than a year, regardless of age (59).

• Forty-three percent of blacks and 36% of whites under age 15 delayed contraceptive use for more than a year. Among 18- to 19-year-old women, 27% of blacks and 12% of whites delayed contraceptive use for more than a year (59).

• Although white and Hispanic males are more likely than blacks to use condoms at first intercourse, more blacks than whites used a condom at most recent intercourse (109).

The 1982 National Survey of Family Growth found noteworthy differences between subgroups of Hispanic 15- to 19-year-old females with respect to the proportion who are sexually active (47).

• Overall, 42% of 15- to 19-year-old Hispanic females have had sexual intercourse. Sixty-nine percent of Cuban, 56% of Central/South American, 41% of other Hispanic, 40% of Puerto Rican, and 39% of Mexican American adolescent females are sexually active (47).

Hispanic women under the age of 20 are more likely than whites to have had a live birth. Fewer are sexually active, but those who are fail to use contraceptives and are less likely to obtain an abortion than white adolescent women (20).

Rates of childbearing among women under 20 years of age are higher among Mexican-American adolescents (38 per 1,000) than Puerto Rican adolescents (30 per 1,000) (39).

Summary and Implications

As children become adolescents, they face increasingly serious health threats that are primarily social rather than medical in origin. Motor vehicle deaths, suicide, homicide, and depression are all major problems for adolescents as a whole. As this chapter has shown, there is clear evidence that some adolescents are more at risk than others for particular health threats, based on their family income, sex, race, ethnicity, or age.

Youth in poverty are more at risk for being in fair or poor health, for abuse and neglect, and for a variety of psychosocial and health risks associated with poverty, such as early, unintended pregnancy, dropping out of school, and other high-risk activities. Adolescent girls are more at risk than boys for abuse and neglect and for eating disorders; boys are more at risk for heavy involvement with alcohol and other drugs. White adolescents are more likely than black adolescents to die of motor vehicle injuries and suicide, and to experiment with and engage in heavy use of drugs, alcohol, and cigarettes. However, death from homicide, drowning, fire, and cancer, as well as rates of sexually transmitted diseases, pregnancy, and childbirth, are all greater among black adolescents than among whites. Older adolescents are more likely than younger adolescents to die or engage in heavy use of alcohol, tobacco, and drugs. Younger adolescents, however, are more likely to begin experimenting with alcohol and tobacco and to delay or fail to use contraceptives effectively, thereby increasing their risk of sexually transmitted diseases and pregnancy.

It is important that prevention and intervention programs targeting adolescents take into account developmental, sex, racial and ethnic, and family income differences that exist among them. The setting and accessibility of health services must be sensitive to these differences and facilitate screening and treatment of adolescents for health problems. Providers must be sensitive to stereotypes about health problems among adolescents and not assume, for example, that problems with substance abuse or sexually transmitted disease are restricted to inner-city, minority populations.

5.

What can be done to improve the health of America's adolescents?

There is no simple or single solution to the complex health problems experienced by adolescents. Their problems include organic and psychological illness as well as "social morbidities," such as adolescent pregnancy, unintentional injury, and consequences of tobacco, alcohol, and drug use. While abnormal organic and psychiatric disorders are sometimes overshadowed by public concern over "social morbidities," they still pose significant health problems for some adolescents. Continued research on these disorders is needed to determine their prevalence, etiology, more effective therapies, and clinical management styles that produce better compliance with medical recommendations.

The social morbidities result from a combination of biological, psychological, and social factors. They must increasingly be viewed in terms of a "prevention model" that promotes environmental and behavioral changes as a means to improve health, and less in terms of a traditional "medical model" in which treatment or rehabilitation of existing problems is the primary issue. This chapter focuses primarily on issues of prevention and reviews what government, private organizations, communities, and organized medicine are doing to improve adolescent health. Cooperative efforts between various groups are also highlighted.

The questions addressed in this chapter are:

1. What are government, private foundations, corporations, and communities doing to improve adolescent health?

2. What is organized medicine doing to improve adolescent health?

3. What research on adolescent health needs to be done?

1. What are government, private foundations, corporations, and communities doing to improve adolescent health?

Although implementation of health strategies usually occurs within communities, establishing health priorities and providing funding mechanisms for programs most often comes from public and private leadership at the national and state levels. The following examples highlight some of the major preventive efforts now under way to improve the health of adolescents.

Public Health Service: Year 2000

The Office of Disease Prevention and Health Promotion (ODPHP) of the Public Health Service, Department of Health and Human Services, has developed "Healthy People 2000," a set of national health goals for the year 2000 (118). Included are objectives for reducing morbidity and mortality rates by the year 2000 for a variety of disorders and conditions. About one third of the objectives are directed at adolescents. The final set of national health objectives will be released in the fall of 1990. Information about this project can be obtained by writing Healthy People 2000, Office of Disease Prevention and Health Promotion, 330 C Street S.W., Room 2132, Washington, DC 20201. The AMA Department of Adolescent Health has received support from ODPHP to promote the health objectives specifically related to adolescents. These activities include publishing the Target 2000 Newsletter and coordinating the National Adolescent Health Promotion Network. Information about activities sur-

rounding the health objectives for adolescents can be obtained by writing the AMA Department of Adolescent Health, 535 N. Dearborn Street, Chicago, IL 60610.

Congressional Commission

The National Commission on Children was established by the U.S. Congress to serve as "a forum on behalf of the children of this nation." The Commission will propose a policy agenda to "improve the opportunities for every American child to achieve his or her full human potential and to enhance the capabilities of families to effectively care for and nurture their children." A report by the Commission is scheduled for release in March 1991. More information can be obtained by writing The National Commission on Children, 1111 18th Street N.W., Suite 810, Washington, DC 20036.

Congressional Reports

The Office of Technology Assessment (OTA), with support from the Carnegie Council on Adolescent Development, is preparing a critical review of the health status of adolescents, the nation's agenda for research and health care services related to adolescents, and factors that endanger or enhance adolescent health. Emphasis is being given to those with special needs, such as rural youth, youth from racial and ethnic minority backgrounds, and economically disadvantaged youth. The final report is due for release in 1990. Additional information can be obtained by writing OTA, U.S. Congress, Washington, DC 20510-8025.

Governor's Association

Members of the National Governor's Association, state legislatures, and other state-level coalitions are developing creative initiatives in adolescent health. Many states are reviewing or have enacted health

Key role played by Dr. C. Everett Koop

A discussion of the role of the federal government in adolescent health would not be complete without acknowledging the efforts of C. Everett Koop, M.D., Sc.D., the recently retired Surgeon General of the United States. During his tenure as Surgeon General, Dr. Koop aggressively addressed preventive efforts in the areas of HIV infection, tobacco use, alcohol-related traffic accidents, and youth with chronic disabilities. During the 1980s, he was the most prominent person at the federal level advocating for the well-being of adolescents. The Surgeon General prepared monographs on the hazards of smoking (115), drunk driving (116), and youth with disabilities (117).

protection laws requiring smoke-free schools. Many states have also increased penalties for driving while under the influence of alcohol and created more stringent regulations of alcohol and tobacco advertising. All states have raised the minimum legal drinking age to 21 years. In Tennessee, alcohol-related motor vehicle fatalities declined by 33% among 15- to 18-year-olds after the legal drinking age was raised to 21 years (42).

Centers for Disease Control

Mandated comprehensive school health education is another example of state efforts to improve adolescent health. The Division of Adolescent and School Health, Centers for Disease Control, in partnership with the Education

Development Center, Inc. (EDC), established the Comprehensive School Health Education Network in 1988 to support state departments of education and health and local school districts in their efforts to provide school health education, particularly with respect to HIV education. To find out more about the network, write Education Development Center, Inc., 55 Chapel Street, Newton, MA 02160.

Carnegie Council

During the past decade, foundations have become especially active in developing new initiatives in adolescent health. The Carnegie Council on Adolescent Development recently released a report, *Turning Points: Preparing American Youth for the 21st Century*, that provides thoughtful recommendations for making junior high and middle schools healthier and less anonymous institutions (33). The Carnegie report concludes that health and fitness are critical to academic performance and need to be improved. Schools could improve student health by:

- Ensuring access to health services through the creation of a "health coordinator" position in every middle school. This person would provide limited medical screening and treatment, refer students to health services outside the school, and coordinate school health education and health-related activities.

- Establishing schools as health-promoting institutions. Health-promoting schools provide smoke-free environments, good nutrition, opportunities for exercise and athletic competition for all students, and a physically safe environment free of violence and weapons.

Robert Wood Johnson Foundation

The Robert Wood Johnson Foundation has funded several programs for high-risk youth, homeless youth, youth who abuse drugs or alcohol, youth who need mental health services, and those who have AIDS (72). The Foundation's School-Based Adolescent Health Care Program, now in its 3rd year, has 24 health centers in 11 states, with services available to nearly 40,000 students. The Foundation also funded the Program to Consolidate Health Services for High-Risk Young People. Between 1982 and 1986, 21 teaching hospitals in 12 states provided a comprehensive package of services to high-risk adolescents in urban areas. Additional information on these programs can be obtained by writing for a copy of "Making Connections: A Summary of Robert Wood Johnson Foundation Programs," available from The Robert Wood Johnson Foundation, College Road, P.O. Box 2316, Princeton, NJ 08543-2316.

Joint Public-Private Initiative

New cooperative efforts between public and private organizations have led to joint funding for projects in designated communities. Such "public-private" ventures frequently generate a community-wide response to broad health problems by sharing financial (and sometimes human) resources. For example, the Ounce of Prevention

Fund, founded in 1982, serves Illinois infants, children, teens, and their families, particularly those "at risk" because of poverty. Public money, funding community-based programs for almost 100,000 Illinois residents, is enhanced by private contributions. The Ounce of Prevention administers several programs, including (a) a state-wide effort to deter adolescent pregnancy and the negative effects of adolescent childbearing and parenting, (b) comprehensive school-based clinics at three Chicago high schools, and (c) a public education and policy project in which staff work with government officials, the media, and other advocacy organizations to increase support for policies and programs serving children and families. The Ounce of Prevention Fund also monitors and evaluates programs on an ongoing basis and, when feasible, uses those findings to initiate new programs in child and adolescent health and development. For further information write Laura Devon Jones, Ounce of Prevention Fund, 188 W. Randolph, Suite 2200, Chicago, IL 60601.

National Center for Youth With Disabilities

The National Center for Youth With Disabilities has been created through a cooperative agreement among the Society for Adolescent Medicine, the Bureau of Maternal and Child Health, and the University of Minnesota. The Center provides information to parents, teachers, and health professionals in order to improve services for disabled youth. The Center publishes a newsletter, *Connections*, and has a computerized list of published material related to youth with disabilities. Additional information can be obtained by writing the National Center for Youth With Disabilities, Adolescent Health Program, University of Minnesota, Box 721-UMHC, Harvard Street at East River Road, Minneapolis, MN 55455.

National Institutes of Health

The National Cancer Institute (84) and the National Heart, Lung, and Blood Institute (110) have funded community-based programs to reduce factors (e.g., sedentary lifestyles, poor diet, and tobacco use) that predispose adolescents to later cardiovascular disease. These programs are unique in their effort to alter personal behavior through coordinated and mutually reinforcing health promotion activities by schools, the media, parents, and community health policy and programs. Interventions are primarily aimed at youth making the transition from elementary to junior high or middle school.

National Collaboration for Youth

The National Collaboration for Youth, a national network of youth-serving organizations, has developed one of the more extensive models of cooperative community activities. This project, entitled *Making the Grade: A Report Card on American Youth*, draws community-level attention to the health problems of adolescents and then coordinates community actions to solve these problems. Since its inception in the summer of 1989, over 400 communities have created local networks to develop programs and activities that promote adolescent health. More information can be obtained by writing Making the Grade, National Collaboration for Youth, 1319 F Street N.W., Suite 601, Washington, DC 20004.

2. What is organized medicine doing to improve adolescent health?

Medical organizations, including medical societies and specialty associations, health maintenance organizations (HMOs), hospitals, and publicly sponsored clinics, have a unique opportunity to improve adolescent health by influencing health policy and promoting the delivery of patient care services. This section provides an overview of major initiatives developed by organized medicine in the areas of clinical services, medical education, and partnership and advocacy. Issues that should receive priority in future efforts are also discussed.

Clinical Services and Access to Care

Access and availability of health services and the content of preventive health care services for adolescents remain priority issues. Access to health care can improve the early detection and management of health problems, thereby reducing the likelihood of more serious consequences of chronic or recurrent disorders and conditions. Organized medicine, health insurance companies, the federal government, and other groups have begun developing programs to improve the delivery of quality health services for adolescents.

Organized medicine is working with other groups and government agencies to develop strategies to increase adolescents' access to quality, confidential, and appropriate health care and social services. Part of this effort focuses on the most vulnerable groups of adolescents, including:

- youth who live in poverty, both in urban and rural areas ;

- youth with physical and mental disorders and disabilities;

- youth who are abused or neglected;

- youth who misuse drugs and alcohol;

- youth who are runaways or homeless;

- youth in correctional facilities;

- youth who lack either private or public sources of health insurance;

- youth from racial or ethnic minority backgrounds.

In 1990, the AMA released its HEALTH ACCESS AMERICA proposal to improve access to affordable, quality health care. Some of the access issues addressed in the 16-point proposal call for (a) major Medicaid reform that would provide uniform adequate benefits to all persons below the poverty level and increase Medicaid reimbursement levels to the Medicare level; (b) requirements that employers provide health insurance for all full-time employees and their families, with tax help to employers that would enable them to afford this health insurance; (c) the creation of state-level risk pools in all states to make available coverage for the medically uninsurable (for whom access to coverage is not available) and for others for whom individual health insurance policies are too expensive and group coverage is not available; and (d) the repeal or overriding of state-mandated benefit laws, to help reduce the cost of health insurance, while assuring through legislation that adequate benefits are provided in all insurance, including self-insurance programs. Additional information can be obtained by writing Health Access America, American Medical Association, 535 N. Dearborn Street, Chicago, IL 60610.

BLUE CROSS/BLUE SHIELD OF WESTERN PENNSYLVANIA, together with PENNSYLVANIA BLUE SHIELD, created the Caring Program for Children. The program provides primary health care coverage to children whose families do not qualify for Medicaid but whose family income is below the federal poverty level. Blue Cross/Blue Shield of Western Pennsylvania used matching contributions from religious groups, businesses, foundations, civic organizations, unions, and individuals to provide health benefits at a cost of $156 per child per year. Since 1985, over 10,000 young people have been covered by this program. The federal Department of Health and Human Services has given Blue Cross of Pennsylvania a grant to replicate the Caring Program for Children nationally. Information about this program can be obtained by writing Caring Program for Children, Fifth Avenue Place, Suite 3012, Pittsburgh, PA 15222.

The U.S. PREVENTIVE SERVICES TASK FORCE has issued a report, the *Guide to Clinical Preventive Services* (119), which contains guidelines to help health practitioners prevent 169 medical disorders and health problems. The guide was published after four years of study and was commissioned by the Office of Disease Prevention and Health Promotion. Although the guide does not address all possible adolescent disorders and conditions, its recommendations offer a first step toward identifying problems that could be addressed when providing health services to adolescents in an office setting.

A more comprehensive set of clinical preventive service recommendations specifically for adolescents should be developed by organized medicine in cooperation with social scientists and health educators. These recommendations should enable clinical practitioners to reinforce appropriate school health messages and help parents and families learn more about how their behavior influences the health practices of their adolescents.

Medical Education

Although specialty medical education in adolescent medicine is strong, many primary care physicians feel that they lack the necessary skills and information to manage the complex biopsychosocial problems of adolescents. Medical organizations should develop creative, new educational

approaches for teaching the principles and techniques of adolescent health care to nonspecialists who see the majority of adolescents in office practices.

Greater involvement of medical students and residents in community field experiences would increase physician sensitivity to the broad nature of adolescent health problems. Valuable field experiences could include working with schools, drug rehabilitation programs, correctional facilities, or volunteer groups that sponsor adolescent health programs, such as health hot lines and mentoring programs.

Education modules could be developed for entire office-based medical practices that include the medical, clerical, and nursing staff. The modules would sensitize all office staff to the needs and concerns of adolescents and develop their skills when dealing with adolescents. The goals of this approach would be increased utilization of medical services by adolescents, greater satisfaction with medical services, and increased compliance by adolescents.

THE AMERICAN ACADEMY OF CHILD AND ADOLESCENT PSYCHIATRY recently completed Project Prevention: An Intervention Initiative. This interdisciplinary effort educates psychiatrists and other health professionals about risk factors and intervention strategies for the prevention of mental health disorders and alcohol and drug abuse. The project report can be found in the monograph, *Prevention of Mental Disorders, Alcohol and Other Drug*

Use in Children and Adolescents (95).

THE AMERICAN ACADEMY OF PEDIATRICS provides an educational newsletter, *Adolescent Health Update: A Clinical Guide for Pediatricians.* Each issue includes information on topics related to the practice of adolescent medicine as well as a list of selected resources for professionals and families. The AAP is also involved in The Adolescent Wellness Program, a joint effort with Health Learning Systems, Inc., and Lederle Laboratories to educate pediatricians about adolescent wellness (including, for example, issues of depression, alcohol and substance use, and sexuality). Information about these programs can be obtained by writing American Academy of Pediatrics, 141 Northwest Point Boulevard, P.O. Box 927, Elk Grove Village, IL 60009-0927.

THE AMERICAN COLLEGE OF OBSTETRICS AND GYNECOLOGY recently published a two-volume guide entitled *Adolescent Sexuality: Guides for Professional Involvement.* The guide offers a wide range of materials that can be used in lectures and presentations on adolescent sexuality and family life education. Included are articles, fact sheets, references, slides, sample handouts, and supplementary material. The guide can be purchased from the ACOG Distribution Center, P.O. Box 91180, Washington, DC 20090 (item No. AA106, parts 1 and 2).

Partnership and Advocacy

Because most adolescent health problems cut across medicine, education, juvenile justice, and social service, the development and dissemination of successful programs require interdisciplinary cooperation and coordination. Although much has been done on behalf of adolescents, many recent initiatives have had a limited impact because they were developed and implemented without the support and input of others working in the same area. Organized medicine must continue to develop partnerships with the many groups involved in adolescent health. More effective advocacy and use of resources result from a strong unified voice.

The AMA and the NATIONAL ASSOCIATION OF STATE BOARDS OF EDUCATION (NASBE), with support from the CENTERS FOR DISEASE CONTROL, are cosponsoring the National Commission on the Role of the School and the Community in Improving Adolescent Health. The purpose of the Commission is to raise national consciousness about the need for educational and health reforms, as well as to motivate communities to reform, invest in, and reinforce school efforts. The report prepared by the Commission is scheduled for release during the summer of 1990. Plans to implement the Commission's recommendations will follow the call to action. Additional information can be obtained by writing either the AMA Department of Adolescent Health, 535 N. Dearborn Street, Chicago, IL 60610, or NASBE, 1012 Cameron Street, Alexandria, VA 22314.

In 1988, the AMA established the AMA ADOLESCENT HEALTH COALI-

TION, consisting of 31 organizations involved in adolescent health. The members of the coalition represent medical specialty societies, government agencies, private foundations, and membership organizations in the health and social service professions. The Coalition provides a vehicle for disseminating information about adolescent health and discussing major issues and initiatives in the area.

Many specialty and state medical societies have successfully advocated for comprehensive health education curricula and prevention programs in unintentional injury, adolescent drug use, unintended pregnancy, and other areas of adolescent health.

Physician-school partnerships

Both nationally and locally, medical groups have successfully advocated for and participated in programs that enhance adolescent health through a close collaboration with schools. The AMA has developed three programs that directly involve physicians with elementary and high school students.

The Natural Science Ambassador Project places young physicians in classrooms to discuss the importance of science in daily life and encourage students to consider health-related careers. Ten states are participating in the project. Further information can be obtained from either the Division of Biomedical Science or the Young Physician Section of the AMA.

AIDS Education: Medical Students Respond trains medical students to provide AIDS education to adolescents. Students from 36 medical schools have participated in the program and have provided AIDS education to over 40,000 adolescents. Information about this program can be obtained by writing the Medical Student Section of the AMA.

The AMA Youth HIV Education Project is a 5-year national program funded by the Division of Adolescent and School Health, Centers for Disease Control. The program trains physicians to support educators teaching HIV and AIDS information to adolescents. Further information about the project can be obtained by writing the Youth HIV Education Project, American Medical Association, 535 N. Dearborn Street, Chicago, IL 60610.

THE AMERICAN ASSOCIATION OF NEUROLOGICAL SURGEONS and the CONGRESS OF NEUROLOGICAL SURGEONS sponsor a National Health and Spinal Cord Injury Prevention Program in 35 states. The program includes a presentation and discussion in high schools about spinal cord injuries. It also includes follow-up activities on the local level, public education programs, and a legislative educational program. Further information can be obtained by writing National Head and Spinal Cord Injury Prevention Program of the AANS/CNS, 22 S. Washington Street, Park Ridge, IL 60068.

THE AMERICAN COLLEGE OF OBSTETRICS AND GYNECOLOGY (ACOG) and the AMERICAN ACADEMY OF FAMILY PHYSICIANS (AAFP) with support from the AMA AUXILIARY are sponsoring a public service program to combat adolescent pregnancy. The campaign uses radio and TV public service announcements in English and Spanish, featuring adolescents who have had unintended pregnancies. Information can be obtained by writing the American College of Obstetrics and Gynecology, Office of Public Information, 409 12th Street S.W., Washington, DC 20024-2188.

The AMERICAN ACADEMY OF PEDIATRICS is involved with the national "Healthy Children" program, funded by the ROBERT WOOD JOHNSON FOUNDATION. The program offers nonfinancial assistance to help communities provide health services to all "children who need them, and to do so at reduced cost through imaginative and efficient use of resources already available in the community" (2). Further information can be obtained by writing the American Academy of Pediatrics, 141 Northwest Point Boulevard, P.O. Box 927, Elk Grove Village, IL 60009-0927.

Better organization and coordination of resources is critically needed at the national, state, and local levels. The development of a coordinating council in the federal government to monitor funding and public policy related to adolescent health should be considered. In addition, organized medicine should also promote and participate in state- and community-level coordinating committees consisting of public and private groups involved in health, education, youth service, advocacy, and policy making.

Organized medicine will continue its role and expand its vigilance to ensure that adolescents receive the health education and health services they need to become healthy and productive adults. In the future, organized medicine is likely to become increasingly involved in issues related to (a) adolescents' access to health care services (e.g., Medicaid coverage, services to underserved youth, availability of school-based health centers, drug testing of students, and confidentiality issues), (b) the coordination and integration of health, education, and social services for adolescents, and (c) preventive services for adolescents.

3. What research on adolescent health needs to be done?

Although major strides have been made during the past decades in understanding the developmental process and health problems associated with adolescence, much more needs to be learned about how physical, emotional, and social factors influence behavior and health, as well as how to apply existing knowledge.

A national research agenda on adolescent health should be developed that is based in part on the federal "Healthy People 2000" health objectives for the nation.

Efforts should be expanded to evaluate the effectiveness of various strategies designed to meet the needs of different groups of adolescents depending on their age, racial and ethnic background, and family income. Research efforts should extend to understanding better the factors that contribute to a healthy transition through adolescence.

Organized medicine, in partnership with other groups, should coordinate existing and future research efforts that would enhance the assessment and monitoring of adolescent health. This might include, for example, a national periodic survey on the incidence, prevalence, and severity of chronic medical conditions and psychiatric disorders among adolescents, access to and utilization of health services, adolescent risk-taking behavior, and other topics to be determined by various experts in adolescent health and survey research. Part of this effort should include the development of consistent age categories across various surveys as well as improving health surveillance systems.

Much research to date has studied categorical issues in health care, such as drug abuse, adolescent pregnancy, and delinquency. However, it is important that research explore the common roots of these problems and the interplay among them.

Given the nature of adolescent health problems, research efforts must increasingly become interdisciplinary and involve collaboration between experts in medicine and the social sciences.

Summary and Implications

A comprehensive program to improve the health of America's youth will require active involvement and commitment by all sectors of society. A first step in this direction is for organizations representing medical and health professionals, educators, and volunteer groups working with adolescents to develop an active agenda in adolescent health for their membership. Increased federal and state action is also needed, including the passage of regulations directed at access to care and health promotion and protection. Ongoing commitments are required from foundations and corporations.

A second step toward improving adolescent health is to disseminate this information and coordinate efforts. This process would enhance advocacy for the health needs of adolescents and produce a more proactive, stronger response to the urgent problems described in previous chapters. Working together, a new beginning for America's adolescents can be forged.

Bibliography

1 Adams, P. F., & Hardy, A. M. (1989). *Current estimates from the national health interview survey, 1988.* Vital and Health Statistics, Series 10, No. 173 (DHHS Publication No. 89-1501). Hyattsville, MD: National Center for Health Statistics.

2 American Academy of Pediatrics. (1989). *Child health care: AAP research update, No. 5.* Elk Grove Village, IL: American Academy of Pediatrics.

3 American Medical Association. (1988). *Reference guide to policy and official statements.* Chicago: American Medical Association.

4 AMA Board of Trustees. (1986). Alcohol: Advertising, counter-advertising, and depiction in the public media. *Journal of the American Medical Association, 256,* 1485-1488.

5 AMA Council on Scientific Affairs. (1987, December). *Report A: Firearms as a public health problem in the United States: Injuries and deaths* (p. 243). Chicago: American Medical Association.

6 AMA Council on Scientific Affairs. (1989, June). *Information report: Recognition of childhood sexual abuse as a factor in adolescent health issues.* Chicago: American Medical Association.

7 AMA Council on Scientific Affairs. (1989). Providing medical services through school-based health programs. *Journal of the American Medical Association, 261,* 1939-1942.

8 AMA Council on Scientific Affairs. (1989). Health status of detained and incarcerated youth. *Journal of the American Medical Association, 263,* 987-991.

9 AMA House of Delegates. (1971, June). *Report I: Teenage pregnancy* (p. 56). Chicago: American Medical Association.

10 AMA House of Delegates. (1971, June). *Report 82: Family planning* (p. 295). Chicago: American Medical Association.

11 AMA House of Delegates. (1973, June). *Resolution 44: Alternatives to therapeutic abortion* (Vol. 2, p. 329). Chicago: American Medical Association.

12 AMA House of Delegates. (1983, December). *Resolution 65: Opposition to HHS regulations on contraceptive services to minors* (p. 291). Chicago: American Medical Association.

13 AMA House of Delegates. (1986, June). *Resolution 46: Support of a tobacco-free society* (p. 368). Chicago: American Medical Association.

14 AMA House of Delegates. (1986, December). *Resolution 114: Media advertising and public service announcements regarding contraception and safe sexual practices* (p. 413). Chicago: American Medical Association.

15 AMA House of Delegates. (1986, December). *Resolution 122: Teenage pregnancy* (p. 415). Chicago: American Medical Association.

16 AMA House of Delegates. (1988, June). *Report NNN: Drug abuse in the United States: A policy report.* Chicago: American Medical Association.

17 AMA House of Delegates. (1989, December). *Resolution 110: Promoting illegal consumption of alcoholic beverages on college campuses.* Chicago: American Medical Association.

18 AMA House of Delegates. (1989, December). *Report X: AMA HIV policy update.* Chicago: American Medical Association.

19 American School Health Association, Association for the Advancement of Health Education, & Society for Public Health Education, Inc. (1989). *The national adolescent student health survey: A report on the health of America's youth.* Oakland, CA: Third Party Publishing Company.

20 Aneshensel, C. S., Fielder, E. P., & Becerra, R. M. (1989). Fertility and fertility-related behavior among Mexican-American and non-Hispanic white female adolescents. *Journal of Health and Social Behavior, 30,* 56-76.

21 Aral, S. O., Schaffer, J. E., Mosher, W. D., & Cates, W., Jr. (1988). Gonorrhea rates: What denominator is most appropriate? *American Journal of Public Health, 78,* 702-703.

22 Athas, C. (1990). National Association of Anorexia Nervosa and Associated Disorders. Highland Park, IL (personal communication, January 26, 1990).

23 Bachman, J. G., Johnston, L. D., & O'Malley, P. M. (1986). *Monitoring the future: Questionnaire responses from the nation's high school seniors, 1986.* Ann Arbor: University of Michigan.

24 Bachmann, G. A., Moeller, T. P., & Benett, J. (1988). Childhood sexual abuse and the consequences in adult women. *Obstetrics and Gynecology, 71,* 631-642.

25 Baker, S. P., O'Neill, B., & Karpf, R. S. (1984). *Injury fact book.* Lexington, MA: Lexington Books.

26 Bezilla, R. (Ed.). (1988). *The Gallup study on America's youth 1977-1988.* Princeton, NJ: The Gallup Organization.

27 Blane, H. T., & Hewitt, L. E. (1977). *Alcohol and youth: An analysis of the literature, 1960-75* (NIAAA Contract No. ADM-281-75-0026). Springfield, VA: National Technical Information Service.

28 Blum, R. (1987). Contemporary threats to adolescent health in the United States. *Journal of the American Medical Association, 257,* 3390-3395.

29 Blum, R.W. (Ed.). (1989). *Chronic illness and disabilities in childhood and adolescence.* Orlando, FL: Grune & Stratton.

30 Breeling, J. L. (1986). Alcohol and the driver. *Journal of the American Medical Association, 255,* 522-527.

31 Buckley, W. E., Yesalis, C. E., Friedl, K. E., Anderson, W. A., Streit, A. L., & Wright, J. E. (1988). Estimated prevalence of anabolic steroid use among male high school seniors. *Journal of the American Medical Association, 260,* 3441-3445.

32 Bureau of Justice Statistics. (1988). *Bureau of Justice Statistics annual report, fiscal 1987*. Washington, DC: U.S. Government Printing Office.

33 Carnegie Council on Adolescent Development. (1989). *Turning points: Preparing American youth for the 21st century*. Report of the Task Force on Education of Young Adolescents. New York: Carnegie Corp.

34 Centers for Disease Control. (1988, November). Trends in human immunodeficiency virus infection among civilian applicants for military service—United States, October 1985-March 1988. *Morbidity and Mortality Weekly Report, 37*, 677-679.

35 Centers for Disease Control. (1988, December). HIV-related beliefs, knowledge and behaviors among high school students. *Morbidity and Mortality Weekly Report, 37*, 717-721.

36 Centers for Disease Control. (1989, November). *HIV/AIDS surveillance report*. Atlanta: Centers for Disease Control.

37 Clayman, C. B. (Ed.). (1989). *The American Medical Association encyclopedia of medicine*. New York: Random House.

38 Cross, A. W. (1985). Health screening in schools: Part II. *The Journal of Pediatrics, 107*, 653-661.

39 Darabi, K. F., & Ortiz, V. (1987). Childbearing among young Latino women in the United States. *American Journal of Public Health, 77*, 25-28.

40 Darnton, N. (1989). Committed youth. *Newsweek*, July 31, 1989.

41 Davis, A. J., & Emans, S. J. (1989). Human papilloma virus infection in the pediatric and adolescent patient. *The Journal of Pediatrics, 115*, 1-8.

42 Decker, M. D., Graitcer, P. L., & Schaffner, W. (1988). Reduction in motor vehicle fatalities associated with an increase in the minimum drinking age. *Journal of the American Medical Association, 260*, 3604-3610.

43 DeKeseredy, W. S. (1988). Woman abuse in dating relationships: The relevance of social support theory. *Journal of Family Violence, 3*, 1-12.

44 Doege, T. C. (1986). Health effects of smokeless tobacco. *Journal of the American Medical Association, 255*, 1038-1044.

45 Dryfoos, J. (1987). *Youth at risk: One in four in jeopardy*. Unpublished report, Carnegie Corp., New York.

46 DuRant, R. H. (1990). Overcoming barriers to adolescents' access to health care. In Hendee, W. R. (Ed.), *The health of adolescents*. San Francisco: Jossey Bass.

47 DuRant, R. H., Pendergrast, R., & Seymore, C. (in press). Sexual behavior among Hispanic female adolescents in the United States. *Pediatrics*.

48 Federal Bureau of Investigation. (1987). *Uniform crime reports for the United States*. Washington, DC: U.S. Government Printing Office.

49 Fingerhut, L. A., & Kleinman, J. C. (1989). *Trends and current status in childhood mortality, United States, 1900-85*. Vital and Health Statistics, Series 3, No. 26 (DHHS Publication No. PHS 89-1410). Hyattsville, MD: National Center for Health Statistics.

50 Finkelhor, D. (1987). The sexual abuse of children: Current research reviewed. *Psychiatric Annals, 17*, 233-241.

51 Flaherty, M. (1980). *An assessment of the incidence of juvenile suicide in adult jails, lockups, and juvenile detention centers: A preliminary report*. Washington, DC: Office of Juvenile Justice and Delinquency Prevention.

52 Gallup Organization, Inc. (1989). *The Waste Management, Inc. survey of parent-child dialogue on drug abuse*. Oak Brook, IL: Waste Management, Inc.

53 Gibbs, J. T. (1988). *Young, black and male in America: An endangered species*. Dover, MA: Auburn House Publishing Co.

54 Gibson, P. (1989). Gay male and lesbian youth suicide. In Feinleib, M. R. (Ed.), *Report of the Secretary's Task Force on Youth Suicide* (Vol. 3) (DHHS Publication No. ADM 89-1623). Washington, DC: U.S. Government Printing Office.

55 Gortmaker, S. (1985). Demography of chronic childhood diseases. In Hobbs, N., Perrin, J., & Ireys, H. (Eds.), *Chronically ill children and their families*. San Francisco: Jossey-Bass.

56 Harvey, L. K., & Shubat, S. C. (1989). *Physician and public attitudes on health care issues, 1989 edition*. Chicago: American Medical Association.

57 Henshaw, S. K., Kenney, A. M., Somberg, D., & Van Vort, J. (1989). *Teenage pregnancy in the United States: The scope of the problem and state responses*. New York: Alan Guttmacher Institute.

58 Hofferth, S. L., & Hayes, C. D. (Eds.). (1987). *Risking the future: Adolescent sexuality, pregnancy, and childbearing* (Vol. 1). Washington, DC: National Academy Press.

59 Hofferth, S. L., & Hayes, C. D. (Eds.). (1987). *Risking the future: Adolescent sexuality, pregnancy, and childbearing* (Vol. 2). Washington, DC: National Academy Press.

60 Hofferth, S. L., Kahn, J. R., & Baldwin, W. (1987). Premarital sexual activity among U.S. teenage women over the past three decades. *Family Planning Perspectives, 19*, 46-53.

61 Hughes, D., Johnson, K., Rosenbaum, S., Butler, E., & Simons, J. (1988). *The health of America's children: Maternal and child health data book*. Washington, DC: Children's Defense Fund.

62 Human Services Research Institute. (1985, December). *Summary of data on handicapped children and youth*. Washington, DC: U.S. Department of Education.

63 Institute of Medicine. (1989). *Research on children and adolescents with mental, behavioral, and developmental disorders: Mobilizing a national initiative*. Washington, DC: National Academy Press.

64 Johnson, K. A. (1986). *Building health programs for teenagers*. Washington, DC: Children's Defense Fund.

65 Johnston, L. D., O'Malley, P. M., & Bachman, J. G. (1987). *National trends in drug use and related factors among American high school students and young adults, 1975-86* (DHHS Publication No. ADM 87-1535). Washington, DC: U.S. Government Printing Office.

66 Johnston, L. D., O'Malley, P. M., & Bachman, J. G. (1988). *Illicit drug use, smoking, and drinking by America's high school students, college students, and young adults, 1975-1987* (DHHS Publication No. ADM 89-1602). Washington, DC: U.S. Government Printing Office.

67 Kandel, D. B. (1982). Epidemiological and psychosocial perspectives on adolescent drug use. *Journal of the American Academy of Child Psychiatry, 21,* 328-347.

68 Kandel, D. B., & Logan, J. A. (1984). Patterns of drug use from adolescence to young adulthood: Periods of risk for initiation, continued use, and discontinuation. *American Journal of Public Health, 74,* 660-666.

69 Kandel, D. B., & Raveis, V. H. (1989). Cessation of illicit drug use in young adulthood. *Archives of General Psychiatry, 46,* 109-116.

70 Klein, J. R., & Litt, I. F. (1981). Epidemiology of adolescent dysmenorrhea. *Pediatrics, 68,* 661-664.

71 Krolnick, R. (1989). *Adolescent health insurance status: Analyses of trends in coverage and preliminary estimates of the effects of an employer mandate and Medicaid expansion on the uninsured.* U.S. Congress, Office of Technology Assessment. Washington, DC: U.S. Government Printing Office.

72 Lear, J. G., Swerdlow, J., Lewin, M. E., & Van Wert, J. (1989). *Making connections: A summary of Robert Wood Johnson Foundation Programs for Adolescents.* Princeton, NJ: The Robert Wood Johnson Foundation.

73 Leary, W. E. (1989, May 23). Campus AIDS survey finds threat is real but not yet rampant. *New York Times.*

74 Lewis, D. W., Feldman, M., & Barrengos, A. (1985). Race, health, and delinquency. *Journal of the American Academy of Child Psychiatry, 24,* 161-167.

75 Marks, A., & Fisher, M. (1987). Health assessment and screening during adolescence. *Pediatrics, 80,* 135-158.

76 Meeks, R. L. (1989). *Utilization of Indian Health Service and contract general hospitals, FY 1988 and U.S. non-federal short-stay hospitals, CY 1987.* Rockville, MD: Indian Health Service.

77 Mensch, B. S., & Kandel, D. B. (1988). Dropping out of high school and drug involvement. *Sociology of Education, 61,* 95-113.

78 Millstein, S. G., Irwin, C. E., Jr., & Brindis, C. (1990). Sociodemographic trends and projections in the adolescent population. In Hendee, W. R. (Ed.), *The health of adolescents.* San Francisco: Jossey Bass.

79 Mitchell, J. (1988, November). *Mental health problems of incarcerated youth.* Paper presented at the AMA Working Group on the Health Status of Detained and Incarcerated Youth, Chicago.

80 Moore, K. A. (1988). *Facts at a glance.* Washington, DC: Child Trends, Inc.

81 Moore, K. A. (1989). *Facts at a glance.* Washington, DC: Child Trends, Inc.

82 Moore, K. A., Nord, C. W., & Peterson, J. L. (1989). Nonvoluntary sexual activity among adolescents. *Family Planning Perspectives, 21,* 110-114.

83 Morris, M. W. (1987). Health care: Who pays the bills? *Exceptional Parent, 17,* 38-41.

84 Murray, D. M., Pirie, P., Luepker, R. V., & Pallonew, U. (1989). Five and six-year follow-up results from four seventh-grade smoking prevention strategies. *Journal of Behavioral Medicine, 12,* 207-218.

85 National Center on Child Abuse and Neglect. (1988). *Study findings. Study of national incidence and prevalence of child abuse and neglect: 1988* (Contract No. 105-85-1702). Washington, DC: U.S. Department of Health and Human Services.

86 National Commission Against Drunk Driving (1988). *Youth driving without impairment: A community challenge.* Report on the youth impaired driving public hearings. Washington, DC: National Highway Traffic Safety Administration.

87 National Institute on Drug Abuse. (1987). *Use of selected drugs among Hispanics: Mexican Americans, Puerto Ricans, and Cuban-Americans: Findings from the Hispanic Health and Nutrition Examination Survey.* Rockville, MD: National Institute on Drug Abuse.

88 National Institute on Drug Abuse. (1985). *National household survey on drug abuse: Main findings 1985.* Washington, DC: U.S. Government Printing Office.

89 National Institute on Drug Abuse. (1989). *National household survey on drug abuse: Population estimates 1988* (DHHS Publication No. ADM 89-1636). Washington, DC: U.S. Government Printing Office.

90 National Institute on Drug Abuse. (1989, August). *Highlights of the 1988 national household survey on drug abuse.* Washington, DC: U.S. Government Printing Office.

91 National Mental Health Association. (1989). *Facts: Children with mental disorders.* Alexandria, VA: National Mental Health Association.

92 Neuman, P. A., & Halvorson, P. A. (1983). *Anorexia nervosa and bulimia: A handbook for counselors and therapists.* New York: Van Nostrand Reinhold.

93 Newacheck, P. W. (1989). Adolescents with special health needs: Prevalence, severity, and access to health services. *Pediatrics, 84,* 872-881.

94 Newacheck, P. W., & McManus, M. A. (1989). Health insurance status of adolescents in the United States. *Pediatrics, 84,* 699-708.

95 Office of Substance Abuse Prevention. (1989). Prevention of mental disorders, alcohol, and other drug use in children and adolescents (Monograph 2) (DHHS Publication No. ADM 89-1646). Washington, DC: U.S. Department of Health and Human Services.

96 Pittman, K., & Adams, G. (1988). *Teenage pregnancy: An advocate's guide to the numbers.* Washington, DC: Children's Defense Fund.

97 President's Council on Physical Fitness and Sports. (1986). *National school population fitness survey.* Ann Arbor: University of Michigan.

98 Reiff, G. G., Dixon, W. R., Jacoby, D., Ye, G. X., Spain, C. G., & Hunsicker, P. A. (1986). *The president's council on physical fitness and sports 1985: National school population fitness survey* (DHHS Contract No. 282-84-0086). Ann Arbor: University of Michigan.

99 Remafedi, G. (1989). *Facts about AIDS and gay teenagers.* Minneapolis: University of Minnesota Youth and AIDS Project.

100 Rimsza, M. E., & Niggemann, E. H. (1982). Medical evaluation of sexually abused children: A review of 311 cases. *Pediatrics, 69,* 8-14.

101 Runyan, C. W., & Gerken, E. (1989). Epidemiology and prevention of adolescent injury: A review and research agenda. *Journal of the American Medical Association, 262,* 2273-2279.

102 Rutter, M. (1980). *Changing youth in a changing society: Patterns of adolescent development and disorder.* Cambridge, MA: Harvard University Press.

103 Saxe, L. M., Cross, T., & Silverman, N. (1986). *Children's mental health: Problems and services.* Report by the Office of Technology Assessment. Durham, NC: Duke University Press.

104 Schiffman, J. R. (1989, February 3) Children's wards: Teen-agers end up in psychiatric hospitals in alarming numbers. *The Wall Street Journal,* p. 1.

105 Select Panel for the Promotion of Child Health. (1981). *Better health for children: A national strategy* (Vol. 3) (DHHS Publication No. 79-55071). Washington, DC: U.S. Government Printing Office.

106 Shafer, M. A., Irwin, C. E., & Sweet, R. L. (1982). Acute salpingitis in the adolescent female. *Journal of Pediatrics, 100,* 339-350.

107 Shafer, M. A., & Moscicki, A. B. (1990). Sexually transmitted diseases in adolescents. In Hendee, W. R. (Ed.), *The health of adolescents.* San Francisco: Jossey-Bass.

108 Sinaiko, A. R., Gomez-Marin, O., & Prineas, R. J. (1989). Prevalence of "significant" hypertension in junior high school-aged children: The Children and Adolescent Blood Pressure Program. *Journal of Pediatrics, 114,* 664-669.

109 Sonenstein, F. L., Pleck, J. H., & Ku, L. C. (1989). Sexual activity, condom use and AIDS awareness among adolescent males. *Family Planning Perspectives, 21,* 152-158.

110 Stone, E. J., Perry, C. L. D., & Luepkes, R. V. (1989). Synthesis of cardiovascular behavioral research for youth health promotion. *Health Education Quarterly, 16,* 155-169.

111 Terney, R., & McLain, L. G. (1990). The use of anabolic steroids in high school students. *American Journal of Diseases of Children, 144,* 99-103.

112 U.S. Congress, Office of Technology Assessment. (1990). *Indian adolescent mental health* (special report OTA-H-446). Washington, DC: U.S. Government Printing Office.

113 U.S. Department of Education. (1988). *Youth indicators, 1988: Trends in the well-being of American youth.* Washington, DC: U.S. Government Printing Office.

114 U.S. Department of Health and Human Services. (1989). *Indian Health Service: Trends in Indian health.* Washington, DC: U.S. Government Printing Office.

115 U.S. Department of Health and Human Services. (1989). *Reducing the health consequences of smoking: 25 years of progress.* Report of the Surgeon General (DHHS Publication No. CDC 89-8411). Washington, DC: U.S. Government Printing Office.

116 U.S. Department of Health and Human Services. (1989). *Surgeon General's Working Conference on Drunk Driving: Proceedings.* Washington, DC: U.S. Government Printing Office.

117 U.S. Department of Health and Human Services. (1989). *Growing up and getting medical care: Youth with special health care needs: A summary of conference proceedings.* National Center for Networking Community-Based Services, Child Development Center. Washington, DC: Georgetown University.

118 U.S. Public Health Service. (1989). *Promoting health/preventing disease: Year 2000 objectives for the nation* (draft). Washington, DC: Department of Health and Human Services.

119 U.S. Preventive Services Task Force. (1989). *Guide to clinical preventive services: An assessment of the effectiveness of 169 interventions.* Baltimore: Williams & Wilkins.

120 Vermund, S. H., Hein, K., Gayle, H. D., Cary, J. M., Thomas, P. A., & Drucker, E. (1989). Acquired immunodeficiency syndrome among adolescents: Case surveillance profiles in New York City and the rest of the United States. *American Journal of Diseases of Children, 143,* 1220-1225.

121 White, S. T., Loda, F. A., Ingram, D. L., & Pearson, A. (1983). Sexually transmitted diseases in sexually abused children. *Pediatrics, 76,* 16-22.

122 Yamaguchi, K., & Kandel, D. B. (1984). Patterns of drug use from adolescence to young adulthood: II. Sequences of progression. *American Journal of Public Health, 74,* 668-672.

123 Yamaguchi, K., & Kandel, D. B. (1984). Patterns of drug use from adolescence to young adulthood: III. Predictors of progression. *American Journal of Public Health, 74,* 673-681.

124 Zabin, L. S., Kantner, J. F., and Zelnick, M. (1979). The risk of adolescent pregnancy in the first months of intercourse. *Family Planning Perspectives, 11,* 215-222.

125 Zetlin, A. G., & Turner, J. L. (1985). Transition from adolescence to adulthood: Perspectives of mentally retarded individuals and their families. *American Journal of Mental Deficiency, 90,* 570-579.

126 Zill, N., & Rogers, C. C. (1988). *Recent trends in the well-being of children in the United States and their implications for public policy.* In Cherlin, A. (Ed.), *Family change and public policy.* Washington, DC: Urban Institute.

Index